# The Ileoanal Pouch

Janindra Warusavitarne • Zarah Perry-Woodford
Editors

# The Ileoanal Pouch

## A Practical Guide for Surgery, Management and Troubleshooting

Springer

*Editors*
Janindra Warusavitarne
St. Mark's Hospital
Harrow
United Kingdom

Zarah Perry-Woodford
St. Mark's Hospital
Harrow
United Kingdom

ISBN 978-3-319-94384-8 ISBN 978-3-319-94385-5 (eBook)
https://doi.org/10.1007/978-3-319-94385-5

Library of Congress Control Number: 2018956325



This Springer imprint is published by the registered company Springer Nature Switzerland AG
The registered company address is: Gewerbestrasse 11, 6330 Cham, Switzerland

# Contents


1 **The History of the Ileoanal Pouch** . . . . . . 1
John Nicholls and Guy Worley

2 **Patient Selection** . . . . . . 15
Michael Powar and Justin Davies

3 **Pouch Configuration** . . . . . . 31
Antonino Spinelli and Marco Ettore Allaix

4 **Pouch Lengthening Techniques** . . . . . . 37
Elaine Burns and Robin Phillips

5 **Minimally Invasive Pouch Surgery: Tips and Tricks** . . . . . . 45
Nicola Hodges and Janindra Warusavitarne

6 **The Complicated Pouch** . . . . . . 55
Willem A. Bemelman, Karin A. T. G. M. Wasmann,
Christianne J. Buskens, and Pieter J. Tanis

7 **Ileal Pouch Salvage, Pouch Failure and Redo Surgery** . . . . . . 75
Constantinos Simillis and Omar Faiz

8 **Crohn's Disease in the Ileal Pouch Anal Anastomosis: Management Strategies** . . . . . . 91
Jonathan Segal and Ailsa Hart

9 **Microbiology of the Ileoanal Pouch and Managing Pouchitis** . . . . . . 105
Simon McLaughlin

10 **Ileoanal Pouch for Familial Adenomatous Polyposis** . . . . . . 115
Ashish Sinha and Sue Clark

11 **The Role of the Ileoanal Pouch Nurse Practitioner** . . . . . . 131
Zarah Perry-Woodford and Samantha Evans

**12 Optimising Pouch Function Using Biofeedback** . . . . . . . . . . . . . . . . . . 153
Brigitte Collins and Elissa Bradshaw

**13 The Kock Pouch (Continent Ileostomy)** . . . . . . . . . . . . . . . . . . . . . . . . . 161
Bruce D. George and Richard Guy

**14 The Ileorectal Anastomosis in Ulcerative Colitis** . . . . . . . . . . . . . . . . . 173
Pär Myrelid and Disa Kalman

**15 The Lived Experience** . . . . . . . . . . . . . . . . . . . . . . . . . . . . . . . . . . . . . . 187
Scott Clifford, Julia Spanswick, Kenny Graham, and Zarah Perry-Woodford

**Index** . . . . . . . . . . . . . . . . . . . . . . . . . . . . . . . . . . . . . . . . . . . . . . . . . . . 193

# Chapter 1
# The History of the Ileoanal Pouch

**John Nicholls and Guy Worley**

**Abstract** This chapter summarises roughly 100 years of innovation in colorectal surgery. Colectomy was introduced as a treatment for ulcerative colitis in the 1940s, dramatically lowering mortality. Quality of life improved markedly with the introduction in the early 1950s of the spout everted ileostomy. By the 1960s there was general consensus that proctocolectomy with permanent ileostomy was the procedure of choice for ulcerative colitis when surgery was indicated.

In parallel, there had been focus on the avoidance of the permanent ileostomy through procedures such as colectomy with ileorectal anastomosis and to a lesser extent proctocolectomy with 'straight' ileoanal anastomosis. With the introduction in the late 1960s of the continent ileostomy which included a small intestinal reservoir and the simultaneous development of endoanal anastomotic technique, the essential elements of restorative proctocolectomy or the 'pouch operation' were in place. The operation was first carried out in the late 1970s and included a mucosal proctectomy with manual anastomosis. The initial 'S' reservoir was modified to a 'J' in the early 1980s and later to a 'W' to increase capacity. The 'J' configuration has proved most used over time. There have been important technical developments of restorative proctocolectomy in the subsequent decades regarding design, the method of construction of the anastomosis, whether a de-functioning ileostomy is routinely necessary and the use of minimally invasive surgery.

**Keywords** Restorative proctocolectomy · Ileoanal pouch · Development Innovation · Ulcerative colitis · Familial adenomatous polyposis

J. Nicholls (✉) · G. Worley
St. Mark's Hospital, Harrow, UK



J. Warusavitarne, Z. Perry-Woodford (eds.), *The Ileoanal Pouch*,
https://doi.org/10.1007/978-3-319-94385-5_1

## 1.1 Introduction

The Ileal Pouch procedure, also referred to as 'Restorative Proctocolectomy' (RPC) or 'Ileal Pouch-Anal Anastomosis' (IPAA), has for over 40 years afforded patients the option to live without a permanent ileostomy after proctocolectomy. The first ileal reservoir with anastomosis to the anus was performed in 1976, and the publication of the technique and the results in five patients in 1978 [1]. Arriving at this point had followed nearly 70 years of evolution in surgery for ulcerative colitis, detailing innovation in the techniques of appendicostomy, ileostomy, total colectomy, proctocolectomy with ileostomy and then with ileoanal anastomosis with the subsequent inclusion of an ileal reservoir or pouch. The chapter will review the events leading up to the creation of the ileal pouch, and the following major developments in pouch surgery up to the present.

## 1.2 The History of Surgery for Ulcerative Colitis

Developments between 1875 and 1888 [2, 3] led to the characterisation of UC as a specific disease separate to infective colitis and a report from the 1909 Royal Society of Medicine (RSM) meeting on ulcerative colitis reported a mortality rate of 48% for patients admitted to London hospitals with UC [4].

Appendicostomy was the first surgical treatment, developed from 1895 onwards, and this involved bringing the appendix to an opening on the skin in order to infuse irrigations, vaccines and serums as topical treatment of the colonic mucosa (Fig. 1.1).

Ileostomy to defunction the large bowel was described by Brown of St Louis in 1913 [5] and became the most used operation over the 1920s and 1930s. The positive effects of resting the large bowel were offset by the high mortality of ileostomy

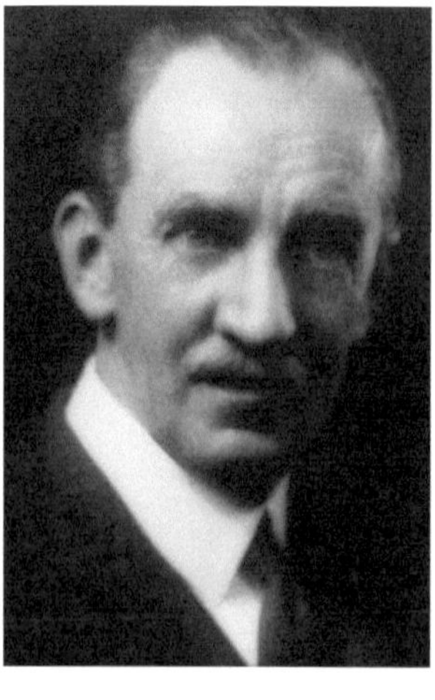

**Fig. 1.1** JP Lockhart Mummery. ("Reproduced with permission from St. Mark's Hospital, Harrow.")

which was around 30% in severely ill patients often with profound hypoalbunimaemia. It was not clear when to operate on patients who were only suffering mild or moderate symptoms, as described in the Royal Society of Medicine (RSM) 1944 presidential address to the Section of Proctology given by Mr Rupert Corbett of St Bartholomew's Hospital, London [6].

In the same era, surgeons were beginning to experiment with surgical removal of the diseased large bowel. Cattell (Fig. 1.2) at the Lahey Clinic, USA, reported 12 patients undergoing colectomy in 1929 with only one death [7]. The strategy of defunctioning by ileostomy changed with the seminal publication of Gavin Miller (Fig. 1.3) and colleagues from Montreal in 1947 who reported the results of 20 patients with severe colitis treated by colectomy with preservation of the rectal stump without any surgical death [8].

Removing the colon and forming an ileostomy had a much reduced mortality than ileostomy alone and by the 1950s the staged approach of colectomy and ileostomy with subsequent removal of the rectum began to take hold. By 1953 Cattell presented a series of 267 patients with a mortality rate from colectomy down to 5%, establishing colectomy as an effective treatment for UC [9].

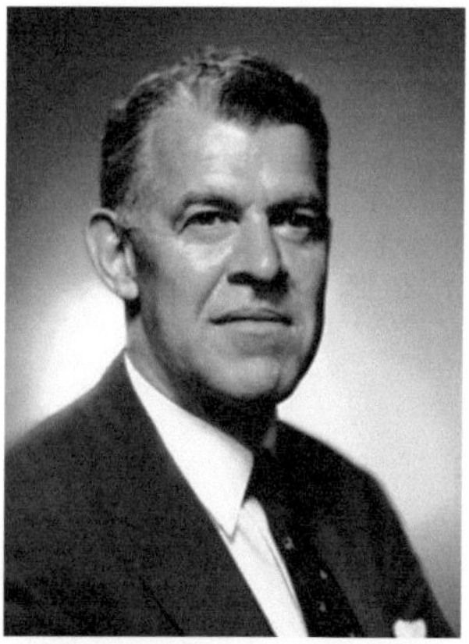

**Fig. 1.2** R Cattell. ("Reproduced from the author's private collection.")

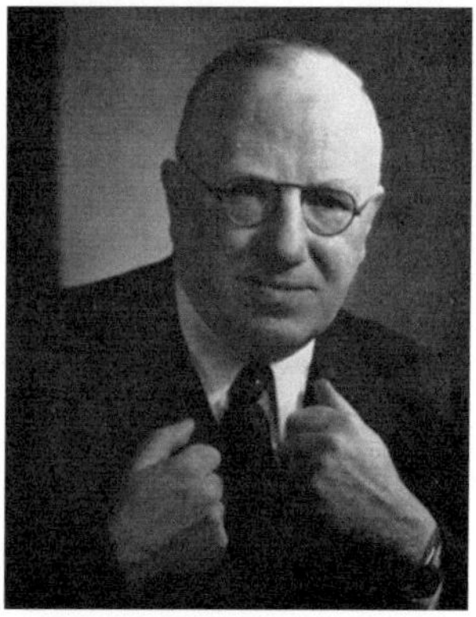

**Fig. 1.3** CG Miller. ("Reproduced with permission from the Royal College of Surgeons of England.")

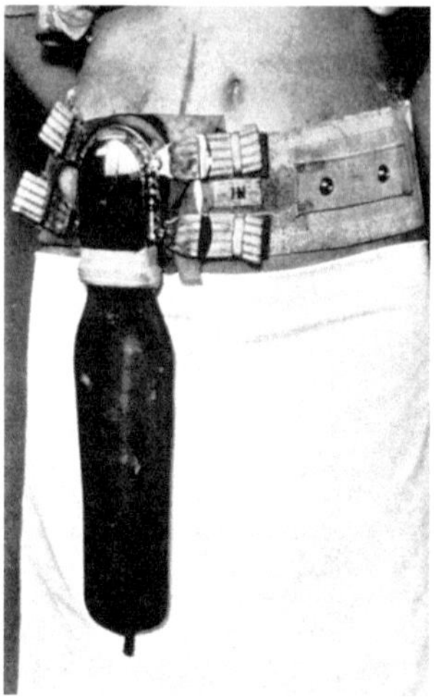

**Fig. 1.4** Early ileostomy appliance

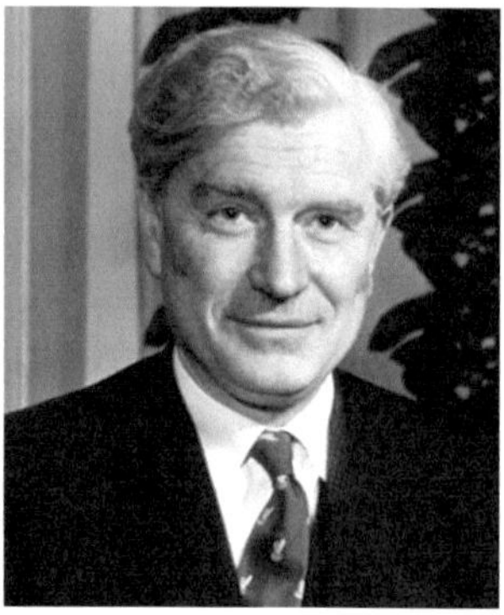

**Fig. 1.5** BN Brooke. ("Reproduced with permission from the Royal College of Surgeons of England.")

The resulting permanent ileostomy presented great practical difficulty for the patient mainly due to the primeval design of the early ileostomy appliance (Fig. 1.4). Various surgical techniques were described to improve quality of life of the patient with an ileostomy, but were not successful until the description by Brooke (Fig. 1.5) in 1952 [10] of the everted ileostomy which created a spout away from the skin edge.

During the first Bipartite meeting of the American Society of Proctology and the Section of Proctology of the Royal Society of Medicine held in London in 1959 [11] proctocolectomy with permanent ileostomy was regarded as the operation of choice for ulcerative colitis when surgery became necessary despite a surgical revision rate of the ileostomy at 5 years of about 10%.

## 1.3 Ileostomy Avoidance

### *1.3.1 Colectomy with Ileorectal Anastomosis*

Owing to the difficulty of managing a permanent ileostomy, some surgeons in the 1940s and 1950s developed ileostomy avoiding procedures. Devine in the 1940s [12] and then Aylett [13] nearly 20 years later, had trialled staged approaches to joining the small bowel to the rectum to form an ileorectal anastomosis after colectomy. Owing to the presence of rectal inflammation as part of the pathology of UC nearly 50% of patients were left with poor bowel function due to the persisting inflammation and the risk of malignant transformation [14] requiring conversion to proctectomy with permanent ileostomy in about one third of cases [15]. Colectomy with ileorectal anastomosis is nevertheless still an option today for carefully selected patients.

### *1.3.2 Restorative Proctocolectomy*

Complete proctocolectomy with ileoanal anastomosis was first described by Nissen (Fig. 1.6) in 1933 in a 12-year-old boy with polyposis, who was continent after the procedure [16]. In 1947 Ravitch and Sabiston rekindled interest in restorative surgery when they published a series of 22 procedures in dogs where the remaining small bowel was joined to the anus forming an 'ileoanal anastomosis'. The mortality of the dogs was high, mostly because of pelvic sepsis, but the procedure was performed successfully in two human patients reported in 1948 [17].

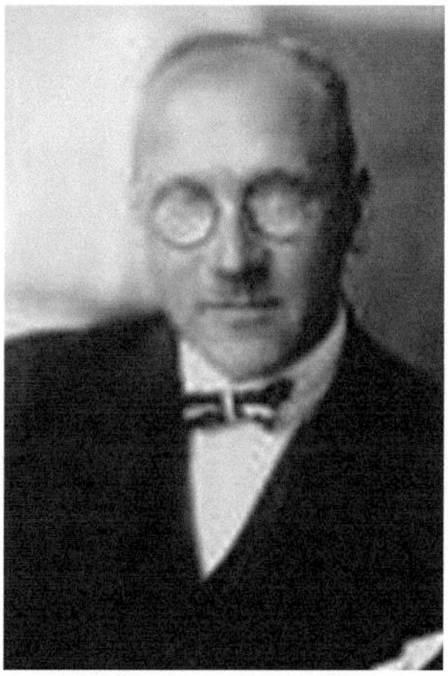

**Fig. 1.6** R Nissen. (https://commons.wikimedia.org/wiki/File:Bundesarchiv_Bild_183-R45871,_Prof._Dr._Ferdinand_Sauerbruch.jpg)

Over the next 10 years a few surgeons carried out what later became known as proctocolectomy with 'straight' ileoanal anastomosis, but a review of the published results by Valiente and Bacon in 1955 [18] revealed high frequency and urgency of defaecation in many cases. Bacon, who contributed so much to colorectal surgery, felt this was due to a lack of rectal reservoir capacitance. He and Valiente carried out experimental reservoir construction in dogs by folding the small bowel on itself to increase capacity. Two out of their seven dogs survived, and the frequency of defaecation was reduced to 2–6 per day. The high mortality discouraged adoption of this procedure in surgical practice, as was commented on by Turnbull who was Chairman of the Department of Colon and Rectal Clinic at the Cleveland Clinic at the time; "…somewhere in the future someone may perhaps solve this problem. I think that it is in the dream stage at the present time".

Originally aiming for bladder replacement after cystectomy, Kock during the 1960s developed a small bowel reservoir which he then applied to the permanent ileostomy created by proctocolectomy to form a 'continent ileostomy' [19]. He constructed a nipple valve by the intussusception of the terminal ileal segment into the reservoir which was closed by intra-abdominal pressure to render the ileostomy continent. Evacuation was effected by the insertion of a catheter via the ileostomy into the reservoir.

Mucosectomy of the lower rectum had been described by both Devine and Peck [20, 21]. This allowed removal of the inflamed mucosa while leaving the rectal muscular wall, enabling an anastomosis between the ileum and the anal canal having removed the proximal disease prone tissue. These technical developments set the scene for the combination of total proctocolectomy with ileoanal anastomosis with the addition of an ileal reservoir to optimise bowel function. The operation was first carried out by at the London Hospital in 1976 by Parks (Fig. 1.7) and subsequently at St. Mark's Hospital. The technique was published in 1978 as 'Proctocolectomy without ileostomy for the treatment of ulcerative colitis', with the results of the first five patients treated [1]. Restorative Proctocolectomy (RPC) has given patients the option to live without a permanent ileostomy after proctocolectomy and remains the standard operation for most patients with ulcerative colitis requiring surgery. It is also applicable to many patients with familial adenomatous polyposis and rarely to some with large bowel cancer and functional bowel disease.

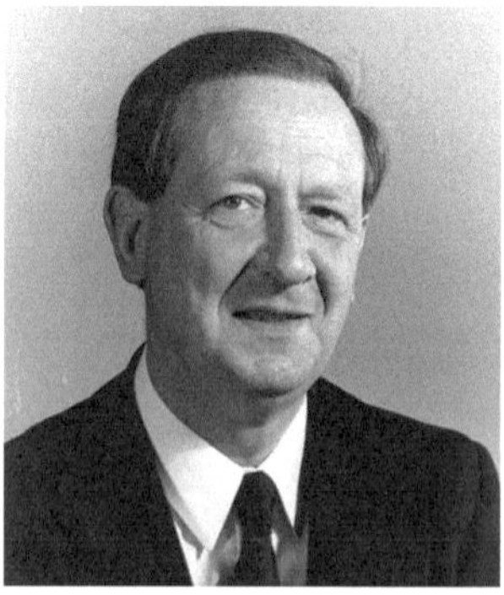

**Fig. 1.7** AG Parks. ("Reproduced from the author's private collection.")

### 1.3.3 Polyposis Syndromes

Selected patients with FAP, Lynch syndrome, Peutz-Jeghers and Juvenile polyposis have undergone RPC. In FAP adenoma formation in a Kock pouch was reported by Beart et al. in 1982 [22] and these lesions were subsequently found in the ileoanal pouch [23, 24].

## 1.4 Restorative Proctocolectomy Since 1978

### 1.4.1 Early Clinical Results

Of the 759 cases presented in a Symposium in 1986 there was only one post-operative death, but there were rates of pelvic sepsis between 8% and 22% and ileoanal anastomotic stricture of 10%. The frequency of defaecation at 6 months after an 'S' or a 'J' pouch construction was five to six times per 24 h, with nocturnal evacuation in 25% of patients [25]. The next decade saw the publication of the results of the first 10 years experience of St. Mark's Hospital (Fig. 1.8) [26], large series from the Mayo (Fig. 1.9) [27] and Cleveland Clinics (Fig. 1.10) [28], Hopital Saint Antoine, Paris,) (Fig. 1.11) [29], Gothenborg where a Kock pouch with ileo-anal anastomosis was favoured (Fig. 1.12) [30] and Mount Sinai Hospital Toronto (Fig. 1.13) [31].

Inflammation in the Kock ileal reservoir had been reported in 1975 [32] and in 1986 pouch inflammation after restorative proctocoloectomy was described in detail with an overwhelming prevalence in UC over FAP [33]. An early review of 'pouchitis' was published in 1990 [34] which offered a definition of the condition. This was followed in 1994 by publication of a pouchitis activity index scoring system developed by Sandborn et al. at the Mayo Clinic [35]. Pouchitis was shown to be amenable to antibiotics and also to probiotic treatment [36, 37].

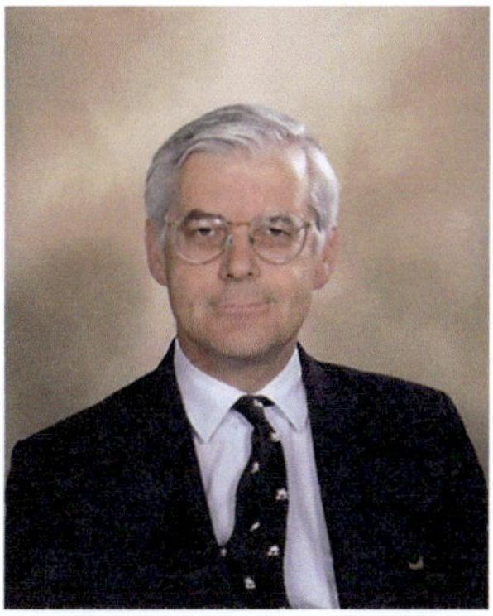

**Fig. 1.8** RJ Nicholls

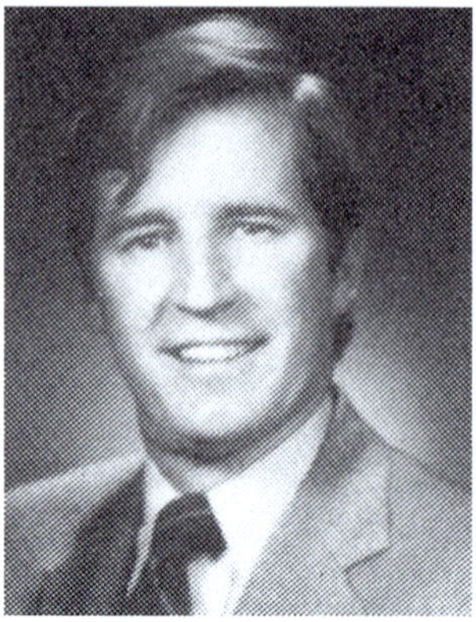

**Fig. 1.9** RR Dozois

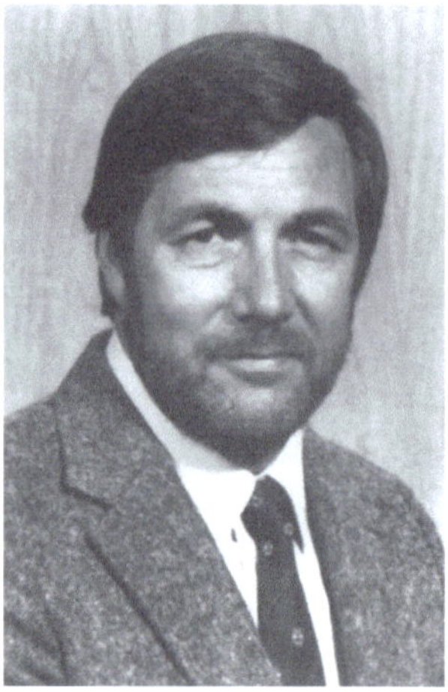

**Fig. 1.10** VW Fazio

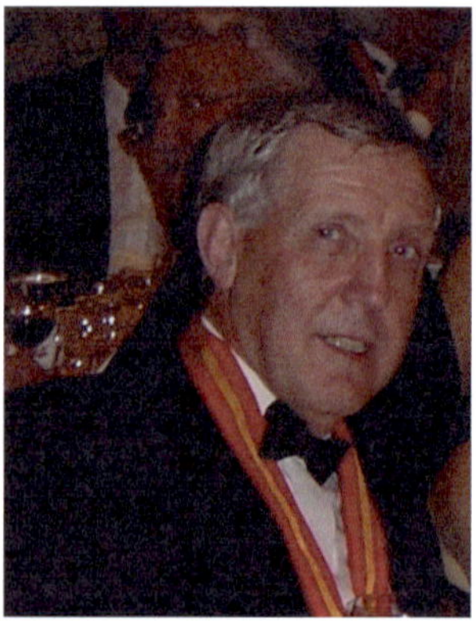

**Fig. 1.11** R Parc

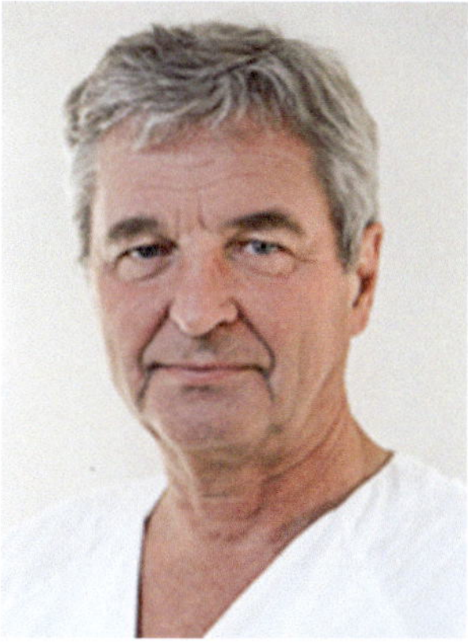

**Fig. 1.12** T Oresland. (http://www.med.uio.no/klinmed/personer/vit/tomor/index.html)

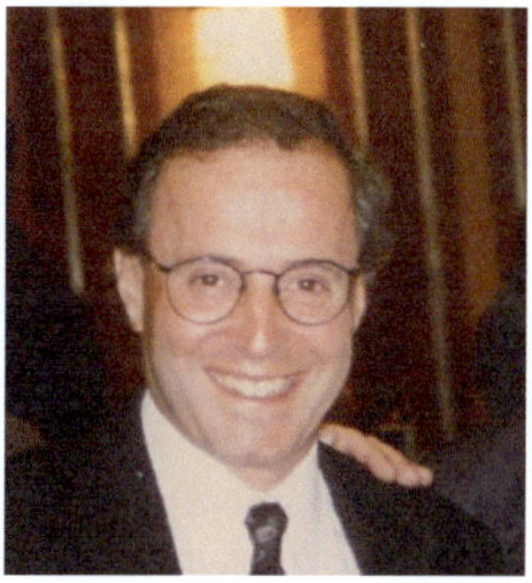

**Fig. 1.13** Z Cohen

A fall in female fecundability was first reported by Olsen et al. in 2001 who showed it to be reduced after RPC to less than 50% of the normal population [38], but not after colectomy with ileorectal anastomosis [39]. Many authors have since confirmed this observation. There is recent evidence that laparoscopic may be associated with a lower incidence of infertility than open surgery [40, 41].

## 1.5 Technical Developments

### *1.5.1 Pouch Design*

The different ileal pouch configurations were described in the early years between 1978 and the mid 1980s. The original 'S' pouch required 60% of patients to catheterise the pouch to empty, due to the long distal ileal limb from the pouch to the anus. This was almost completely avoided by the J-pouch described by Utsunomiya et al. (Fig. 1.14) in 1980 [42] and the need for anal catheterisation to evacuate the pouch became very uncommon. Function was further improved and the operation

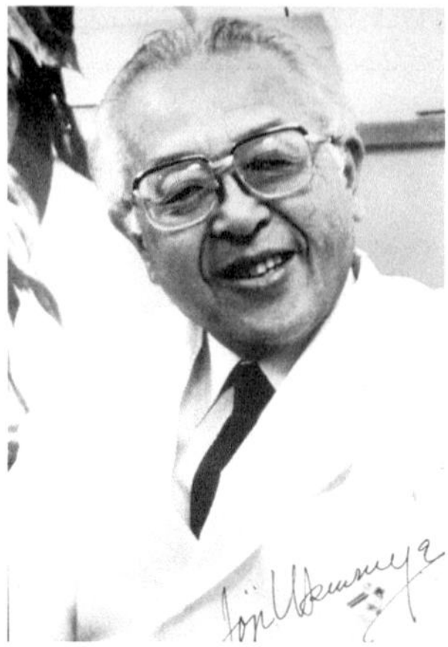

**Fig. 1.14** J Utsunomiya. (http://www.cancer.or.jp/outline.html rights belong to BCPF)

made easier by the removal of the rectum with ileoanal anastomosis performed directly between the pouch and the anorectal junction just above the dentate line.

An inverse relationship between capacity and frequency of defaecation was reported in 1986 [43] as it had earlier for the straight ileoanal neorectum [44]. For this reason a larger reservoir, the W-pouch, was designed to ensure a pouch of adequate capacitance [45]. Fonkalsrud had developed another design referred to as the 'H-pouch' [46]. The 'J' pouch is the simplest to create and now the most popular. Meta-analysis of the three different designs did not find any difference in the short term outcome, but confirmed the greater need for catheterisation in 'S' pouches, which are now almost obsolete. A greater requirement for anti-diarrhoeal medication was found for 'J' than for 'W' pouches, but a randomised trial comparing 'J' and 'W' configurations with 68% of participants followed up to 8.7 years showed that the 'W' pouch advantage was only evident at 1 year. By 9 years there was no difference between the two forms of reconstruction, and so the 'J' pouch became established as the most used pouch design [47, 48].

### *1.5.2 The Ileoanal Anastomosis*

The ileoanal anastomosis was originally constructed manually using the technique described by Parks. It included a mucosectomy to remove the most distal part of the disease. The initially long rectal cuff became shorter and with the increasing use of stapling devices the anastomosis was increasingly performed mechanically [49]. A manual anastomosis gives greater precision of height, is less likely to stricture and allows mucosectomy to remove almost all the inflamed colorectal mucosa. In contrast a stapled anastomosis is technically simpler and for this reason has become the more frequently used technique. It may furthermore result in less stretching of the anal sphincter. A meta-analysis showed a similar short-term outcome with either technique although there was better night time continence in the stapled group but less chance of leaving inflamed mucosa after manual anastomosis [50].

### 1.5.3 Defunctioning Stoma

There are conflicting data on whether a defunctioning ileostomy reduces anastomotic leakage, but it is commonly accepted that the septic sequelae are reduced [51, 52]. There is however a significant morbidity of stoma formation and closure operations of 20–40%, the majority being local complications or ileus, and anastomotic leakage of 4–5%. This rate of comorbidity has led some surgeons to argue the case for avoiding de-functioning ileostomy in all but selected high-risk cases [53].

### 1.5.4 Minimally Invasive Techniques

In one of the first reports of the use of multiport laparoscopy in performing RPC, Santoro et al. [54] described five patients operated on between 1993 and 1996 without any intra-or post-operative complications. Bemelman et al. reported a series of 16 patients in 2001 in whom quality of life and function were no different to a group of 19 patients having open surgery [55]. Subsequent techniques have included single-incision laparoscopic surgery (SILS) and transanal minimally invasive surgery (TAMIS) [56, 57]. A meta-analysis of laparoscopic vs open pouch surgery including 27 comparative studies of 2428 patients [58] showed longer operating times and slightly shorter inpatient stay. There was a lower incidence of wound infection and intra-operative blood loss with no difference in failure and improved function.

### 1.5.5 Long Term Outcome and Failure

Failure rates initially were reported to be around 5% but follow up over several years showed that there was a steady unremitting rise of failure with time [59]. Over a 20 year period a failure of 6% at 20 years was reported at the Mayo Clinic [60]. Failure was considerably higher in a UK national audit of ten centres performing RPC with rates of around 20% at 20 years [61]. Over this period there was an increase in anal soiling, although frequency of defaecation remained the same. The learning curve related to failure at the Cleveland Clinic was estimated to be around 23 cases for trainees [62].

Mechanical failure due to stricture formation at the IAA, a retained rectal stump or threatened failure due to sepsis have been treated by salvage surgery with satisfactory results, particularly in non-septic cases [63–69].

## References

1. Parks AG, Nicholls RJ. Proctocolectomy without ileostomy for ulcerative colitis. Br Med J. 1978;2:85–8.
2. Wilks S, Moxon W. Lectures on pathological anatomy. 2nd ed. London: J&A Churchill; 1875.

3. White H. On simple ulcerative colitis and other rare intestinal tumours. Lancet. 1888;131:1130–1.
4. Cammeron H, Rippman CH. Statistics of ulcerative colitis from London hospitals. Proc R Soc Med. 1909;2:100.
5. Brown J. The value of complete physiological rest of the large bowel in the treatment of certain ulcerative and obstructive lesions of this organ. Surg Gynecol Obstet. 1913;16:610.
6. Corbett CR. A review of the surgical treatment of chronic ulcerative colitis. Proc R Soc Med. 1945;38:277.
7. Cattell R. New type of ileostomy for chronic ulcerative colitis. Surg Clin North Am. 1939;19:629–35.
8. Miller CG, Ripstein CB, Tabah EG. The surgical management of ulcerative colitis surgery. Gynecol Obstet. 1949;88:351–8.
9. Cattell R. Discussion on the surgery of ulcerative colitis. Proc R Soc Med. 1953;46:1021.
10. Brooke BN. The management of an ileostomy. Lancet. 1952;260:102–4.
11. Warner E, Taylor S. Meeting of the Section of Proctology of the Royal Society of Medicine with the American Proctological Society. London June 29-July 1. Proc R Soc Med. 1959;52(Suppl. 3):31.
12. Devine H. Method of colectomy for desperate cases of ulcerative colitis. Surg Gynecol Obstet. 1943;76:136.
13. Aylett SO. Three hundred cases of diffuse ulcerative colitis treated by total colectomy and Ileo-rectal anastomosis. Brit med J. 1966;1:1001–5.
14. Newton CR, Baker WN. Comparison of bowel function after ileorectal anastomosis for ulcerative colitis and colonic polyposis. Gut. 1975;16:785–91.
15. Hawley PR. Ileorectal anastomosis. Br J Surg. 1985;72(S1):s75–6.
16. Nissen R. Sitzungsberichte aus Chirurgischen Gesellschaften Berliner Gesellschaft für Chirurgie. Zentralbl Chir. 1933;60:888.
17. Ravitch MM, Sabiston DC. Anal ileostomy with sphincter preservation in patients requiring total colectomy for benign conditions. Surgery. 1948;24:170–87.
18. Valiente MA, Rey H, Rico P, Bacon HE. Construction of pouch using 'pantaloon' technic for pull-through of ileum following total colectomy. Am J Surg. 1955;90:742–50.
19. Kock NG. Intra-abdominal 'reservoir' in patients with permanent ileostomy. Arch Surg. 1969;99(2):223–31.
20. Devine J, Webb R. Resection of the rectal mucosa, colectomy, and anal ileostomy with normal continence. Surg Gynecol Obstet. 1951;92:437–42.
21. Peck DA, German JD, Jackson FC. Rectal resection for benign disease: a new technic. Dis Colon Rectum. 1966;9:363–6.
22. Beart RWJ, Fleming CR, Banks PM. Tubulovillous adenomas in a continent ileostomy after proctocolectomy for familial polyposis. Dig Dis Sci United States. 1982;27(6):553–6.
23. Wu JS, McGannon EA, Church JM. Incidence of neoplastic polyps in the ileal pouch of patients with familial adenomatous polyposis after restorative proctocolectomy. Dis Colon Rectum United States. 1998;41(5):552–7.
24. Parc YR, Olschwang S, Desaint B, Schmitt G, Parc RG, Tiret E. Familial adenomatous polyposis: prevalence of adenomas in the ileal pouch after restorative proctocolectomy. Ann Surg. 2001;233(3):360–4.
25. Dozois RR, Goldberg SM, Rothenberger DA, Utsunomiya J, Nicholls RJ, Cohen Z, Hulten L, Moskowitz RL, Williams NS. Symposium restorative proctocolectomy with ileal reservoir. Int J Colorectal Dis. 1986;1:2–19.
26. Setti-Carraro P, Ritchie JK, Wilkinson KH, Nicholls RJ, Hawley PR. The first 10 years' experience of restorative proctocolectomy for ulcerative colitis. Gut. 1994;35:1070–5.
27. Pemberton JN, Kelly KA, Beart RW, Dozois RR, Wolff BG, Ilstrup DM. Ileal pouch-anal anastomosis for chronic ulcerative colitis: long term results. Ann Surg. 1987;206:504–13.
28. Fazio VW, O'Riordain MG, Lavery IC, Church JM, Lau P, Strong SA, et al. Long-term functional outcome and quality of life after stapled restorative proctocolectomy. Ann Surg. 1999;230:575.

29. Tiret E, Kartheuser A, Legrand M, Penna C, Parc R. Ileo-anal pouch anastomosis: results in ulcero-hemorrhagic rectocolitis and in familial adenomatous polyposis. Acta Gastroenterol Belg Belgium. 1990;53(4):423–9.
30. Oresland T, Fasth S, Nordgren S, Hulten L. The clinical and functional outcome after restorative proctocolectomy. A prospective study in 100 patients. Int J Colorectal Dis. 1989;4:50–6.
31. Cohen Z, McLeod RS, Stern H, Grant D, Nordgren S. The pelvic pouch and ileoanal anastomosis procedure. Surgical technique and initial results. Am J Surg. 1985;150:601–7.
32. Philipson B, Brandberg A, Jagenburg R, Kock NG, Lager I, Ahren C. Mucosal morphology, bacteriology, and absorption in intra-abdominal ileostomy reservoir. Scand J Gastroenterol. 1975;10:145–53.
33. Moskowitz RL, Shepherd NA, Nicholls RJ. An assessment of inflammation in the reservoir after restorative proctocolectomy with ileoanal ileal reservoir. Int J Colorectal Dis. 1986;1:167–74.
34. Madden MV, Farthing MJ, Nicholls RJ. Inflammation in ileal reservoirs: 'pouchitis. Gut. 1990;31:247–9.
35. Sandborn WJ, Tremaine WJ, Batts KP, Pemberton JH, Phillips SF. Pouchitis after ileal pouch-anal anastomosis: a pouchitis disease activity index. Mayo Clin Proc. 1994;69:409–15.
36. Gionchetti P, Rizzello F, Helwig U, Venturi A, Lammers KM, Brigidi P, et al. Prophylaxis of pouchitis onset with probiotic therapy: a double-blind, placebo-controlled trial. Gastroenterology. 2003;124:1202–9.
37. Heuschen UA, Autschbach F, Allemeyer EH, Zollinger AM, Heuschen G, Uehlein T, et al. Long-term follow-up after ileoanal pouch procedure: algorithm for diagnosis, classification, and management of pouchitis. Dis Colon Rectum United States. 2001;44:487–99.
38. Olsen KO, Joelsson M, Laurberg S, Oresland T. Fertility after ileal pouch-anal anastomosis in women with ulcerative colitis. Br J Surg. 1999;86:493–5.
39. Olsen KO, Juul S, Bulow S, Jarvinen HJ, Bakka A, Bjork J, et al. Female fecundity before and after operation for familial adenomatous polyposis. Br J Surg. 2003;90:227–31.
40. Bartels SAL, D'Hoore A, Cuesta MA, Bensdorp AJ, Lucas C, Bemelman WA. Significantly increased pregnancy rates after laparoscopic restorative proctocolectomy: a cross-sectional study. Ann Surg. 2012;256:1045–8.
41. Beyer-Berjot L, Maggiori LL, Birnbaum D, Lefevre JHJH, Berdah SS, Panis Y. A total laparoscopic approach reduces the infertility rate after ileal pouch-anal anastomosis: a 2-center study. Ann Surg. 2013;258:275–82.
42. Utsunomiya J, Iwama T, Imago M, Matsuo S, Sawai S, Yaegashi K, Hirayama R. Total colectomy, mucosal proctectomy and ileo-anal anastomosis. Dis Colon Rectum. 1980;23:459–66.
43. Nicholls RJ, Pezim ME. Restorative proctocolectomy with ileal reservoir for ulcerative colitis and familial adenomatous polyposis: a comparison of three reservoir designs. Br J Surg. 1985;72:470–4.
44. Heppell J, Kelly KA, Phillips SF, Beart RW Jr, Telander RL, Perrault J. Physiologic aspects of continence after colectomy, mucosal proctectomy, and endorectal ileo-anal anastomosis. Ann Surg. 1982;195:435–43.
45. Nicholls RJ, Lubowski DZ. Restorative proctocolectomy: the four loop (W) reservoir. Br J Surg. 1987;74:564–6.
46. Fonkalsrud EW. Endorectal ileoanal anastomosis with isoperistaltic ileal reservoir after colectomy and mucosal proctectomy. Ann Surg. 1984;199:151–7.
47. Lovegrove RE, Heriot AG, Constantinides V, Tilney HS, Darzi AW, Fazio VW, Nicholls RJ, Tekkis PP. Meta-analysis of short-term and long-term outcomes of J, W and S ileal reservoirs for restorative proctocolectomy. Colorectal Dis. 2007;9:310–20.
48. McCormick PH, Guest GD, Clark AJ, Petersen D, Clark DD, Stevenson AR, Stitz R. The ideal ileal-pouch design: a long-term randomized control trial of J- vs W-pouch construction. Dis Colon Rectum. 2012;55:1251–7.
49. Heald RJ, Allen DR. Stapled ileo-anal anastomosis: a technique to avoid mucosal proctectomy in the ileal pouch operation. Br J Surg. 1986;73:571–2.

50. Lovegrove RE, Constantinides VA, Heriot AG, Athanasiou T, Darzi A, Remzi FH, Nicholls RJ, Fazio VW, Tekkis PP. A comparison of hand-sewn versus stapled Ileal Pouch Anal Anastomosis (IPAA) following proctocolectomy. Ann Surg. 2006;244:18–26.
51. Wong NY, Eu KW. A defunctioning ileostomy does not prevent clinical anastomotic leak after a low anterior resection: a prospective, comparative study. Dis Colon Rectum. 2005;48(11):2076–9.
52. Weston-Petrides GK, Lovegrove RE, Tilney HS, Heriot AG, Nicholls RJ, Mortensen NJ, Fazio VW, Tekkis PP. Comparison of outcomes after restorative proctocolectomy with or without defunctioning ileostomy. Arch Surg. 2008;143:406–12.
53. Gignoux BM, Dehni N, Parc R, Tiret E. Ileal pouch anal-anastomosis without covering ileostomy. Gastroenterol Clin Biol. 2002;26:671–4.
54. Santoro E, Carlini M, Carboni F, Feroce A. Laparoscopic total proctocolectomy with ileal J pouch-anal anastomosis. Hepatogastroenterology Greece. 1999;46(26):894–9.
55. Dunker MS, Bemelman WA, Slors JF, van Duijvendijk P, Gouma DJ. Functional outcome, quality of life, body image, and cosmesis in patients after laparoscopic-assisted and conventional restorative proctocolectomy: a comparative study. Dis Colon Rectum. 2001;44:1800–7.
56. Leo CA, Samaranayake S, Perry-Woodford ZL, Vitone L, Faiz O, Hodgkinson JD, et al. Initial experience of restorative proctocolectomy for ulcerative colitis by transanal total mesorectal rectal excision and single-incision abdominal laparoscopic surgery. Colorectal Dis. 2016;18:1162–6.
57. Borstlap WAA, Harran N, Tanis PJ, Bemelman WA. Feasibility of the TAMIS technique for redo pelvic surgery. Surg Endosc. 2016;30:5364–71.
58. Singh P, Bhangu A, Nicholls RJ, Tekkis P. A systematic review and meta-analysis of laparoscopic vs open restorative proctocolectomy. Colorectal Dis. 2013;15:e340–51.
59. Tulchinsky H, Hawley PR, Nicholls J. Long-term failure after restorative proctocolectomy for ulcerative colitis. Ann Surg. 2003;238(2):229–34.
60. Hahnloser D, Pemberton JH, Wolff BG, Larson DR, Crownhart BS, Dozois RR. Results at up to 20 years after ileal pouch–anal anastomosis for chronic ulcerative colitis. Br J Surg. 2007;94(3):333–40.
61. Tekkis PP, Lovegrove RE, Tilney HS, Smith JJ, Sagar PM, Shorthouse AJ, Mortensen NJ, Nicholls RJ. Long-term failure and function after restorative proctocolectomy – a multi-centre study of patients from the UK National Ileal Pouch Registry. Colorectal Dis. 2010;12:433–41.
62. Tekkis PP, Fazio VW, Lavery IC, Remzi FH, Senagore AJ, Wu JS, Strong SA, Poloneicki JD, Hull TL, Church JM. Evaluation of the learning curve in ileal pouch-anal anastomosis surgery. Ann Surg. 2005;241:262–8.
63. Galandiuk S, Scott NA, Dozois RR, Kelly KA, Ilstrup DM, Beart RW Jr, Wolff BG, Pemberton JH, Nivatvongs S, Devine RM. Ileal pouch-anal anastomosis. Reoperation for pouch-related complications. Ann Surg. 1990;212:446–52.
64. Fazio VW, Wu JS, Lavery IC. Repeat ileal pouch-anal anastomosis to salvage septic complications of pelvic pouches: clinical outcome and quality of life assessment. Ann Surg. 1998;228:588–97.
65. Meagher A P, Farouk R, Dozois RR, Kelly KA, Pemberton JH. J ileal pouch-anal anastomosis for chronic ulcerative colitis: complications and long-term outcome in 1310 patients. Br J Surg. 1998;85:800–3.
66. MacLean AR, O'Connor B, Parkes R, Cohen Z, McLeod RS. Reconstructive surgery for failed ileal pouch-anal anastomosis: a viable surgical option with acceptable results. Dis Colon Rectum. 2002;45:880–6.
67. Tulchinsky H, McCourtney JS, Rao KV, Chambers W, Williams J, Wilkinson KH, Nicholls RJ. Salvage abdominal surgery in patients with a retained rectal stump after restorative proctocolectomy and stapled anastomosis. Br J Surg. 2001;88:1602–6.
68. Dehni N, Remacle G, Dozois RR, Banchini F, Tiret E, Parc R. Salvage reoperation for complications after ileal pouch-anal anastomosis. Br J Surg. 2005;92:748–53.
69. Tekkis PP, Heriot AG, Smith JJ, Das P, Canero A, Nicholls RJ. Long-term results of abdominal salvage surgery following restorative proctocolectomy. Br J Surg. 2006;93:231–7.

# Chapter 2
# Patient Selection

**Michael Powar and Justin Davies**

**Abstract** Patient selection, including active patient involvement, is of paramount importance in the setting of ileal pouch-anal anastomosis (IPAA) surgery. In the following chapter, we discuss the indications for surgery and key patient, disease and surgical considerations.

**Keywords** Ileal pouch anal anastomosis · Ileoanal pouch · Inflammatory bowel disease · Dysplasia · Colorectal cancer · Patient selection

Ileal pouch anal anastomosis (IPAA) surgery is a major undertaking for any patient considering it, as well as for the surgical and wider team involved. It is also an operation for quality of life, as there is always an alternative option that likely includes a stoma. Therefore, selecting the correct patient for the procedure, and ensuring their active involvement in the decision-making process, is of paramount importance.

## 2.1 Ulcerative Colitis

Ulcerative colitis is a chronic inflammatory condition that affects the rectum and colon proximally for a variable distance. Although this condition is, in the majority of patients, managed effectively with medication, approximately 1 in 5 patients with ulcerative colitis will require surgery during their lifetime [1]. Furthermore, resection of all disease-prone tissue by means of a proctocolectomy is potentially curative in ulcerative colitis. The natural history of ulcerative colitis dictates the indication for surgery. Within the first year of diagnosis the risk of surgery is high for patients who present with acute severe colitis refractory to medical therapy. In contrast, within 5 years of diagnosis, the indication for surgery is more often due to steroid

M. Powar · J. Davies (✉)
Cambridge Colorectal Unit, Addenbrooke's Hospital, Cambridge University Hospitals NHS Foundation Trust, Cambridge, UK

 
J. Warusavitarne, Z. Perry-Woodford (eds.), *The Ileoanal Pouch*,
https://doi.org/10.1007/978-3-319-94385-5_2

dependent or intractable disease. From a decade after diagnosis, dysplasia or the development of cancer may play an increasing role in the need for proctocolectomy. The cumulative probability of colectomy from the time of diagnosis was 13.1% at 5 years, 18.9% at 10 years and 25.4% at 20 years in a population-based cohort in Minnesota [2]. The indications for surgery in ulcerative colitis can be acute or elective.

### 2.1.1 Acute

Acute severe ulcerative colitis, defined by Truelove and Witt, is a potentially life-threatening condition [3, 4]. Intravenous corticosteroids remain the mainstay of conventional therapy. Patients are best managed by a multi-disciplinary approach between gastroenterologists and colorectal surgeons. Close monitoring and evaluation of the patient should take place and complications such as toxic megacolon, perforation or severe gastrointestinal haemorrhage necessitate immediate colectomy. Objective assessment of the patient and clinical course should take place after 72 h of intravenous corticosteroids. Treatment options including colectomy should be discussed with patients failing to respond satisfactorily. Second line "rescue" therapy with intravenous Cyclosporin or Infliximab may be considered. If no improvement is seen with 7 days of medical treatment, then colectomy is indicated, to minimise the increased peri-operative complications associated with delayed surgery [5]. It is important to appreciate that, even in patients with acute severe colitis who exhibit a good initial response to medical therapy, the eventual need for colectomy can range from 20% to 80% [6–8].

Successful outcomes of restorative proctocolectomy with IPAA in selected patients with acute "moderate" fulminant colitis have been reported [9, 10]. However, due to the patient's physiological, pharmacological (steroid use) and nutritional state, pouch surgery, in general, should be avoided in the acute setting. Instead, the goal of surgery is to resect the bulk of diseased bowel, with reliable minimal morbidity, whilst preserving future potential restorative options for the patient once they have recovered. Sub-total colectomy with formation of end ileostomy is safe, effective and reproducible at addressing these goals [11]. A laparoscopic sub-total colectomy and end ileostomy has been shown to be safe, feasible and has potential clinical benefits of reduced wound and intra-abdominal sepsis and shorter hospital stay compared with an open approach [11, 12]. Furthermore, there are data to suggest that patients undergoing laparoscopic surgery initially have a reduced interval to subsequent IPAA and ileostomy closure [13]. Evidence to guide optimal surgical management of the rectosigmoid stump following sub-total colectomy for acute severe colitis is unclear [14–16]. Options include a closed intra-peritoneal stump, exteriorization of a mucus fistula or securing the closed stump in an extra-peritoneal subcutaneous position. The latter option potentially confers the advantage of reduced pelvic sepsis in the event of stump dehiscence as well as facilitating identification and pelvic dissection at subsequent surgery (along with preservation of the inferior mesenteric artery at the time of initial subtotal colectomy). Transanal drainage using a Foley catheter may also aid decompression of the rectum in the immediate postoperative period [17].

Clearly the colectomy specimen should be examined microscopically to confirm the pathological diagnosis. In patients with a pathologically confirmed diagnosis of ulcerative colitis, a subsequent completion proctectomy and IPAA may be considered in order to remove the remaining diseased rectum and restore intestinal continuity at a later date.

### 2.1.2 Elective

Surgery is indicated in the elective setting when the patient has medically refractory disease, develops steroid-dependence, the side effects of medication significantly impair the patient's quality of life or dysplasia or cancer is present.

### 2.1.3 Intractable Disease

Intractability is the most common indication for surgery in chronic ulcerative colitis. Symptoms may be refractory to optimal medical management. Alternatively, adequate symptom control with intensive medical therapy may be achieved but patients are unable to tolerate side effects or unwilling to accept risks of long term medical treatment.

Proctocolectomy with formation of IPAA has become increasingly popular over the last four decades and is now the most common elective surgical procedure performed in chronic ulcerative colitis. However, panproctocolectomy with permanent end ileostomy should still be considered definitive treatment for patients who elect not to undergo a restorative procedure or who are considered at high risk of pouch failure due to anal sphincter dysfunction, ano-perineal disease or limited physiological reserve from significant co-morbidities [18, 19]. The procedure is safe, effective and curative, allowing the majority of patients to live full and active lives [20]. The mainstay of complications are stoma related but also include small bowel obstruction, perineal wound sinus and bladder and sexual dysfunction [21].

The rationale for restorative proctocoloectomy with IPAA in patients with ulcerative colitis is that excision of the colon and rectum removes disease prone tissue, whilst construction of an ileal pouch restores a "reservoir" and performing a pouch-anal anastomosis re-establishes intestinal continuity with voluntary defaecation. This achieves the desired goal of avoiding a permanent stoma. IPAA can be performed safely with an acceptable morbidity rate (19–27%) and mortality is rare (0.2–0.4%) [22, 23]. The results have been shown to be durable with a quality of life trending towards that of a healthy individual [24–27].

### 2.1.4 Dysplasia/Cancer

Malignancy in ulcerative colitis is multifactorial, with genetic mutations similar to sporadic colorectal cancer, in addition to continued inflammation resulting in cell proliferation, oxidative stress and subsequent dysplasia [28, 29]. However, unlike sporadic cancers, cancers in ulcerative colitis may not follow a sequential step-wise progression from normal epithelium to low grade dysplasia, high grade dysplasia and ultimately invasive malignancy. Despite this, the presence and grade of dysplasia is the current measure used to identify patients at risk of developing cancer [30]. However, a proportion of patients undergoing proctocolectomy have a concomitant colorectal cancer. Over the past three decades, case series have emerged from several centres detailing IPAA procedures in over 200 patients with colorectal cancer [31–40]. Reported functional outcomes and complication rates in cancer patients have been comparable to patients free of malignancy.

There are notable considerations when performing IPAA surgery in this group of patients. It is important not to compromise oncological aspects of the surgical resection to perform a restorative procedure. From a technical perspective, when undertaking a restorative proctocolectomy for benign disease surgeons may preserve the ileocolic artery and perform a "low" ligation of the inferior mesenteric pedicle. To ensure satisfactory nodal harvest, high ligation of vascular pedicles should be performed in patients with colorectal cancer. Surgery for locally advanced right sided colonic tumours may necessitate resection of a significant length of distal ileum and associated mesentery. This may result in difficulties with adequate mesenteric length for the constructed pouch reservoir to be delivered tension-free into pelvis. For rectal cancers, pelvic dissection should proceed in a nerve-sparing mesorectal plane rather than a close rectal dissection to achieve a total mesorectal excision. These technical considerations do not preclude the performance of an IPAA. However, resection of low rectal tumours which do not allow sphincter preservation are clearly not suitable for restorative IPAA surgery.

For patients with locally advanced rectal cancer it is important to consider the need for neo-adjuvant radiotherapy. As the small bowel is particularly sensitive to radiation damage [41], there are obvious concerns regarding creation of an IPAA in a potential radiation field and adverse effects on anastomotic healing and subsequent functional outcome. Within the limited case series of colorectal cancer patients undergoing IPAA there are relatively few patients with rectal cancer with only a fraction treated with radiotherapy [32–40]. Interestingly, the majority of these patients received post-operative adjuvant radiotherapy with a significant proportion developing subsequent pouch failure and excision. In a reported series from Toronto, six patients with rectal cancer who underwent IPAA were potential candidates for radiotherapy [42]. Four patients opted to avoid radiotherapy after appropriate counselling and the remaining two had neoadjuvant therapy.

No patients in this cohort with poorly differentiated or T4 low rectal tumours were offered a restorative procedure. This case series reported on 73 patients undergoing proctocolectomy for colorectal cancer including 39 patients undergoing IPAA and 34 patients undergoing permanent ileostomy. They compared survival outcomes and found no significant difference in overall or disease-free survival in patients undergoing IPAA compared with permanent end ileostomy. Furthermore, there was no significant difference in survival between colon and rectal cancers. A retrospective review of clinical features and oncologic outcomes of 41 patients with rectal cancer who underwent IPAA at the Mayo Clinic in Minnesota identified that in 17% of cases the cancer was detected post-operatively in the pathological specimen [32]. Notably, no patient who received neoadjuvant chemoradiotherapy progressed to a restorative procedure with construction of an IPAA. The majority of patients in this cohort had stage I or II disease, however of note, 89% of the observed recurrences were in patients with stage III and IV disease.

There are a lack of robust data to support an oncologic advantage of mucosectomy and hand-sewn anastomosis over stapled anastomosis in the presence of dysplasia or cancer. Mucosectomy does not guarantee removal of all mucosa and subsequent cancers have been described in both patients with mucosectomy and stapled anastomoses [43]. However, when the indication for surgery is high grade dysplasia of the lower rectum, it would be reasonable to perform a mucosectomy and anastomosis at the dentate line [5].

Several case series have reported a slightly increased pouch failure rate amongst patients with colorectal cancer undergoing IPAA compared with those free of malignancy (10–18%) [32, 33, 35, 42]. The reasons for this are likely to be multifactorial but may be related to cancer cachexia and (neo)adjuvant chemotherapy/radiotherapy treatments which affect tissue healing and subsequent functional outcome.

A further important consideration to guide decision making is the complex and multi-stage nature of IPAA surgery compared with the single stage nature of panproctocolectomy and formation of permanent end ileostomy. Furthermore, approximately one-fifth of ulcerative colitis patients with cancer who undergo IPAA will succumb to metastatic disease [37]. As a consequence, some have advocated a more conservative staged approach with initial performance of colectomy and end ileostomy and subsequent consideration of restorative procedure after an interval of 12 months to ensure there is no early development of local or distant disease recurrence [38]. Metastatic disease is generally considered a contra-indication to performing IPAA. The priority in these patients is timely local and distant disease control, which may involve colectomy, chemotherapy and surgery for metastases. Potential complications related to IPAA surgery may delay or interrupt chemotherapy, adversely affecting the patient's oncological outcome. Therefore, given the quality of life implications, construction of an IPAA may not be deemed appropriate for patients with poor prognosis disease, high risk of cancer recurrence or limited lifespan.

Although the evidence base is not high quality, these data suggest that providing the technical aspects of surgical oncology are adhered to, IPAA can be performed in the setting of colon cancer and upper/mid T1 or T2 rectal cancer. The small number of patients makes it difficult to confidently interrogate the potential adverse effects of neoadjuvant treatment on postoperative pouch complications and function. However, it is the authors practice not to offer IPAA to patients who require neoadjuvant treatment, have a T3/T4 rectal cancer or cancer in the lower one third of the rectum. To optimise outcomes, all patients should be fully staged preoperatively and their case discussed at a multidisciplinary cancer meeting. Furthermore, appropriate patient education and counselling is essential so that the patient understands the oncologic and functional implications and is fully involved in decision making process.

### 2.1.5 *Special Considerations*

Deciding to undergo IPAA is a major decision for any patient. In addition, there will be some particular considerations that the surgical team will wish to factor in to this process. Below, we outline some of these factors, some of which may be modifiable, and thus important to consider in terms of potentially improving surgical outcome.

#### 2.1.5.1 Patient Factors

Age

Historically, IPAA was not offered to elderly patients because of concerns regarding impaired sphincter function following the prolonged anal dilatation required to perform a mucosectomy and hand-sewn IPAA [44]. The advent of the double stapling technique, avoiding prolonged anal dilatation, resulted in several single centre series reporting IPAA in patients aged over 50 years [45–50]. Functional outcomes and long term complication rates in selected patients over 50 are comparable with younger patients [51]. During the first year following IPAA, there was similar daytime stool frequency (5–6 per day) between the two groups but younger patients experienced slightly less nocturnal stool frequency (mean 1.4 v 1.9). At 1 year, incontinence episodes were reported by less than one quarter of patients under 45 years of age compared with approximately half of those aged over 55. Similar long-term functional observations have been seen in patients over 50 with greater than 12 years' follow-up following IPAA [52]. The low cumulative risk of pouch failure was comparable between younger and older patients in this series of 1386 patients. A systematic review of age-stratified studies assessing functional outcomes of IPAA found that although day and night time incontinence rates were significantly higher in older patients at 1 year, function deteriorated with time across all ages, and after 10 years there was no significant difference in incontinence rates between age groups [53]. Dehydration and electrolyte loss was however a significant problem in patients over 65 years of age. Despite these functional differences between younger and older patients, there was no significant difference in the high patient satisfaction rates with IPAA procedure at 10 years following surgery [51].

Disease severity is known to be an important factor in perioperative complications in patients with ulcerative colitis. Possible explanations as to why age may not appear to be associated with increased morbidity include the fact that older patients have less severe disease and more commonly require surgery for dysplasia [48]. Recent interest has focused on frailty, rather than chronological age, as a contributor for surgical risk. Frailty is a state of reduced physiologic reserve reflecting function, cognition, nutrition and co-morbidities [54]. Frailty is associated with increased perioperative morbidity, mortality and length of stay across surgical specialities. The relationship of frailty and age and impact on surgical outcomes and length of stay for patients undergoing IPAA has been examined at the population level using the American College of Surgeons National Surgical Quality Improvement Program database [55]. This analysis identified that older age (>60 years) was associated with a small increase in hospital length of stay (0.8 days) but no significant increase in major complications. Furthermore, frailty trait count was not associated with a significant increase in hospital length of stay or major complications.

Chronological age in isolation should not preclude selection of patients for IPAA. Appreciation of associated co-morbidity, anal sphincter function and patient's mental state should help guide decision making. IPAA is safe and feasible in selected, counselled and well-motivated elderly individuals with appropriate support for the potential functional difficulties that can accompany this procedure [56].

## Obesity

The prevalence of obesity is escalating in the Western world. There is an increasing number of patients with ulcerative colitis being considered for IPAA who are obese [57]. From a technical perspective there are specific challenges of IPAA in obesity. Obese patients often have a shortened small bowel mesentery which has obvious implications for pouch reach for anastomosis as well as traversing the broader abdominal wall from peritoneum to skin for defunctioning ileostomy formation. Obese patients (BMI > 30 kg/m$^2$) experience significantly higher peri-operative and cumulative complications, including wound infections, anastomotic leak and pelvis sepsis [58, 59]. Furthermore, IPAA surgery is associated with significantly increased length of stay and incisional hernia development [60]. Obese patients also exhibit a significantly higher rate of pouch related complications including anastomotic stricture, inflammation (pouchitis and cuffitis) and pouch fistula formation [61].

Increased stricture formation may be related to ischaemia resulting from delivering a thickened, foreshortened pouch mesentery into a deep pelvis. Similarly, the technical challenges of cross stapling the rectum at the pelvic floor may contribute to increased retention of rectal mucosa and subsequent cuffitis. Finally, the difficulty of constructing a low anastomosis in an obese patient may impact the development of pouch fistulae.

A potential surgical strategy for obese patients may include three-stage IPAA, where suitably motivated patients are supported to lose weight prior to undergoing an elective IPAA. Prospective studies to evaluate whether this reduction of BMI correlates with a decreased incidence of pouch related complications would be informative. Pre-operative counselling for obese patients being considered for IPAA should include a frank discussion regarding alternatives including permanent end ileostomy and of the increased rate of postoperative complications.

#### 2.1.5.2 Disease Factors

Medical Therapy

Moderate to high dose steroids (20 mg of prednisolone or greater) are associated with increased short term pouch specific complications (odds ratio 10.2), surgical site infections (odds ratio 7.96) and general infectious complications (odds ratio 5.19) [62]. Prior exposure to azathioprine or mercaptopurine, from a week up to a month before pouch surgery, does not appear to significantly impact short or long term morbidity [63].

The impact of biologic therapy, initiating inhibitors of tumour necrosis factor alpha, on outcomes after pouch surgery remain controversial. Retrospective observational studies from the Mayo and Cleveland Clinics suggest that previous exposure to infliximab (IFX) was associated with an increase in short-term complications following pouch surgery, including anastomotic leak, pouch specific and infectious complications [64, 65]. These findings prompted the authors to propose that patients who had previous IFX treatment may be served by a 3-stage pouch procedure to minimise the risk of inferior outcomes [64]. Reports conflicting this finding have emerged from Belgium, Denmark and the USA, with no increase in morbidity associated with IFX use within 12 weeks of surgery [65–67]. A Dutch study of patients undergoing a single stage pouch procedure (without defunctioning ileostomy) found increased rates of pelvic sepsis in patients previously exposed to IFX [68]. The lack of clarity on the impact of anti-TNF-alpha therapy may be due to most studies being heterogeneous, retrospective and observational, lacking standardized definitions of complications.

Primary Sclerosing Cholangitis

The performance of IPAA in patients with ulcerative colitis and primary sclerosing colitis (PSC) should be considered with caution. A retrospective comparative study of patients with ulcerative colitis both with and without PSC identified an increasingly divergent risk of pouchitis over a 20-year period (65% in PSC group v 28% in non-PSC group) [69]. Furthermore, PSC patients were more likely to experience poor nocturnal pouch function (37% v 2%). However, there were no significant differences in surgical complications, quality of life and sexual function. As such, it is imperative that patients with ulcerative colitis and PSC are appropriately counselled regarding the significant risks of pouchitis and potential for sub-optimal pouch function prior to embarking on pouch surgery.

Indeterminate Colitis and Crohn's Disease

Complications of IPAA surgery, such as pelvic sepsis and fistulae, are higher in patients with indeterminate colitis compared to those with ulcerative colitis [70]. The long term pouch failure rates for patients with indeterminate colitis electing to have IPAA surgery remain higher than for those with ulcerative colitis, and this is likely due to a proportion of patients initially diagnosed with indeterminate colitis subsequently being diagnosed with Crohn's disease. However, careful counselling of the patient does not preclude IPAA surgery in this cohort of patients with indeterminate colitis, as long as the increased risk of complications and subsequent pouch failure is discussed.

Patients with Crohn's disease however, do have a much higher pouch failure rate [71] than those with ulcerative or indeterminate colitis, with failure rates over 50% in most series. Therefore, IPAA surgery is generally not recommended in the setting of Crohn's disease, although some highly motivated patients and surgeons may seek to consider this option in the setting of isolated colonic Crohn's disease in the absence of any other small bowel or perianal involvement.

#### 2.1.5.3 Surgeon Factors

Laparoscopic Surgery

Laparoscopic IPAA has been shown to be feasible and safe in several studies [72, 73]. The adoption of a laparoscopic approach for ulcerative colitis increased by 8.5% each year on review of the NSQIP database from 2005 to 2008 and was associated with lower morbidity and mortality [74]. A Cochrane review in 2009 of over 600 patients found length of stay, complications, reoperation, readmissions and mortality rates for laparoscopic IPAA were not significantly different from an open approach [75]. Patients who have undergone laparoscopic surgery have a significantly higher satisfaction with the cosmetic scar and higher body image scores with similar quality of life outcome measures to those undergoing open IPAA [76].

Retrospective review of two stage pouch procedures has demonstrated that laparoscopic surgery is associated with a shorter interval to closure of ileostomy [77]. Laparoscopic IPAA has been shown to be associated with significantly fewer intraperitoneal and pelvic adhesions as assessed by diagnostic laparoscopy at time of ileostomy closure [78]. In line with this, recent reports also have demonstrated improved preservation of female fecundity following laparoscopic IPAA compared with open procedures [79, 80].

## 2.2 Functional Bowel Disorders

Surgery may be indicated in selected patients with functional bowel disorders characterised by colonic inertia with or without rectal inertia. Resection of part or all the colon has been described as a possible treatment option for chronic constipation since Sir Arbuthnot Lane's paper in 1908 [81]. Colectomy for a more defined group of patients with slow transit constipation was described in the early 1980s [82].

Colectomy with ileo-rectal anastomosis, the commonest procedure performed, peaked in popularity in the 1990s. However, sub-optimal long term outcomes and high complication rates have resulted in its more judicious application subsequently [83, 84]. It is of interest that as a consequence of poor functional outcome, particularly recurrent constipation or diarrhoea and incontinence, up to 28% of patients go on to have a permanent ileostomy fashioned. Further important considerations when embarking on surgery for functional bowel disorders is the presence of idiopathic megacolon or megarectum. A plethora of surgical procedures have been performed in patients with idiopathic megacolon, including segmental and total colectomy, rectal and pelvic floor procedures and stoma formation [85]. Systematic review has identified that colectomy may resect dilated colon but in delivering liquid stool to a potentially dysmotile rectum the patients bowel function can continue to be poor.

In 1988, Nicholls reported on two cases of proctocolectomy with restorative ileoanal reservoir for severe idiopathic constipation [86]. Both patients had persisting constipation following previous colectomy and an excision of the rectum, formation of an ileal reservoir with ileoanal anastomosis was performed. Symptomatic improvement was achieved in both patients with only one exhibiting objective improvements in transit studies and proctography and the other requiring catheterization to evacuate the pouch. Permanent ileostomy was avoided in both patients. Restorative proctocolectomy with IPAA was also applied to a series of 13 patients with functional bowel disorders, including 5 with megacolon and megarectum [87]. Cross-stapling of the megarectum was technically difficult and all of these patients underwent a hand-sewn IPAA of which 2 experienced anastomotic leaks. Mean day pouch stool frequency was 4.8 times and 6 patients experienced night time soiling. The pouch was converted to ileostomy in two patients due to persistent complications and associated poor functional result. The same group subsequently described their experience of IPAA in a series of 14 patients with megacolon and megarectum over 16 years [88]. Eleven of these patients had undergone previous surgery. Functional outcomes at follow-up identified that 12 patients were continent, one patient experiencing minor soiling and frank incontinence in another. Due to persistent symptoms of abdominal pain and bloating, 4 patients were dissatisfied with the outcome and proceed to pouch excision. It is noteworthy that construction of an end ileostomy did not ameliorate the symptoms of abdominal pain and distension in these patients.

Kalbassi and colleagues investigated the technical and functional success of IPAA in patients with slow transit constipation and concomitant rectal inertia. Furthermore, the impact on quality of life was reported in this case series of 15 patients over 7 years [89]. Quality of life questionnaires were used preoperatively and at follow-up with emphasis on physical function, role limitation, social function, pain and general health. All patients had failed long-term conservative therapy and were selected based on normal colonoscopy and anal manometry with abnormal colonic transit and proctography. Significant improvements in quality of life scores were recorded in the categories of physical function, social function, and pain at the first follow-up (1–3 years after surgery) and in all categories at the second follow-up (>3 years after surgery). Two patients underwent pouch excision within 18 months due to persistent and intractable pelvic pain despite satisfactory pouch function.

The limited evidence base comprised of small case series lends difficulty in recommending a clear role for IPAA in functional bowel disorders characterised by severe idiopathic constipation with rectal inertia. Quality of life for certain patients may be improved, but the magnitude of surgery and potential for complications is significant. It is also important to appreciate that in clinic practice, a proportion of patients with functional bowel problems may have pan-enteric dysmotility, eating or psychological disorders, and these will additional factors will adversely affect outcomes. If embarking on IPAA for functional bowel disorders it is imperative that careful selection, with rigorous preoperative assessment and extensive counselling including formal psychological evaluation is performed.

## 2.3 Conclusion

Patient selection is crucial in terms of ensuring best possible patient outcomes in IPAA surgery. Although ulcerative colitis remains the main indication for surgery, other pathologies may occasionally be considered for this surgery, but the importance of multidisciplinary decision making, with active patient involvement, remains key.

## References

1. Carter MJ, Lobo AJ, Travis SP, IBD Section BSoG. Guidelines for the management of inflammatory bowel disease in adults. Gut. 2004;53:V1–16.
2. Samuel S, Ingle SB, Dhillon S, et al. Cumulative incidence and risk factors for hospitalization and surgery in a population-based cohort of ulcerative colitis. Inflamm Bowel Dis. 2013;19:1858–66.
3. Truelove SC, Witts LJ. Cortisone in ulcerative colitis; final report on a therapeutic trial. Br Med J. 1955;2:1041–8.
4. Bernstein CN, Ng SC, Lakatos PL, Moum B, Loftus EV Jr. A review of mortality and surgery in ulcerative colitis: milestones of the seriousness of the disease. Inflamm Bowel Dis. 2013;19:2001–10.
5. Oresland T, Bemelman WA, Sampietro GM, et al. European evidence based consensus on surgery for ulcerative colitis. J Crohns Colitis. 2015;9:4–25.
6. Oshitani N, Kitano A, Matsumoto T, Kobayashi K. Corticosteroids for the management of ulcerative colitis. J Gastroenterol. 1995;30(suppl 8):118–20.
7. Campbell S, Travis S, Jewell D. Ciclosporin use in acute ulcerative colitis: a long-term experience. Eur J Gastroenterol Hepatol. 2005;17:79–84.
8. Moskovitz DN, Van Assche G, Maenhout B, et al. Incidence of colectomy during long-term follow-up after cyclosporine-induced remission of severe ulcerative colitis. Clin Gastroenterol Hepatol. 2006;4:760–5.
9. Ziv Y, Fazio VW, Church JM, Milsom JW, Schroeder TK. Safety of urgent restorative proctocolectomy with ileal pouch- anal anastomosis for fulminant colitis. Dis Colon Rectum. 1995;38:345–9.
10. Harms BA, Myers GA, Rosenfeld DJ, Starling JR. Management of fulminant ulcerative colitis by primary restorative proctocolectomy. Dis Colon Rectum. 1994;37:971–8.
11. Teeuwen PH, Stommel MW, Bremers AJ, van der Wilt GJ, de Jong DJ, Bleichrodt RP. Colectomy in patients with acute colitis: a systematic review. J Gastrointest Surg. 2009;13:676–86.

12. Marceau C, Alves A, Ouaissi M, Bouhnik Y, Valleur P, Panis Y. Laparoscopic subtotal colectomy for acute or severe coli- tis complicating inflammatory bowel disease: a case-matched study in 88 patients. Surgery. 2007;141:640–4.
13. Chung TP, Fleshman JW, Birnbaum EH, Hunt SR, Dietz DW, Read TE, et al. Laparoscopic vs. open total abdominal colectomy for severe colitis: impact on recovery and subsequent completion restorative proctocolectomy. Dis Colon Rectum. 2009;52:4–10.
14. Carter FM, McLeod RS, Cohen Z. Subtotal colectomy for ulcerative colitis: complications related to the rectal remnant. Dis Colon Rectum. 1991;34:1005–9.
15. Gu J, Stocchi L, Remzi F, Kiran RP. Intraperitoneal or subcutaneous: does location of the (colo)rectal stump influence outcomes after laparoscopic total abdominal colectomy for ulcerative colitis? Dis Colon Rectum. 2013;56:615–21.
16. Trickett JP, Tilney HS, Gudgeon AM, Mellor SG, Edwards DP. Management of the rectal stump after emergency sub-total colectomy: which surgical option is associated with the lowest morbidity? Colorectal Dis. 2005;7:519–22.
17. Karch LA, Bauer JJ, Gorfine SR, Gelernt IM. Subtotal colectomy with hartmann's pouch for inflammatory bowel disease. Dis Colon Rectum. 1995;38:635–9.
18. Fazio VW, Tekkis PP, Remzi F, et al. Quantification of risk for pouch failure after ileal pouch anal anastomosis surgery. Ann Surg. 2003;238:605–14.
19. Metcalf AM. Elective and emergent operative management of ulcerative colitis. Surg Clin North Am. 2007;87:633–41.
20. Jimmo B, Hyman NH. Is ileal pouch-anal anastomosis really the procedure of choice for patients with ulcerative colitis? Dis Colon Rectum. 1998;41:41–5.
21. Carlstedt A, Fasth S, Hultén L, Nordgren S, Palselius I. Long- term ileostomy complications in patients with ulcerative colitis and Crohn's disease. Int J Colorectal Dis. 1987;2:22–5.
22. Fazio VW, Ziv Y, Church JM, et al. Ileal pouch-anal anastomoses complications and function in 1005 patients. Ann Surg. 1995;222:120–7.
23. Meagher AP, Farouk R, Dozois RR, Kelly KA, Pemberton JH. J ileal pouch-anal anastomosis for chronic ulcerative colitis: complications and long-term outcome in 1310 patients. Br J Surg. 1998;85:800–18.
24. McIntyre PB, Pemberton JH, Wolff BG, Beart RW, Dozois RR. Comparing functional results one year and ten years after ileal pouch-anal anastomosis for chronic ulcerative colitis. Dis Colon Rectum. 1994;37:303–7.
25. Leowardi C, Hinz U, Tariverdian M, et al. Long-term outcome 10 years or more after restorative proctocolectomy and ileal pouch-anal anastomosis in patients with ulcerative colitis. Langenbecks Arch Surg. 2010;395:49–56.
26. Tiainen J, Matikainen M. Health-related quality of life after ileal J-pouch-anal anastomosis for ulcerative colitis: long-term results. Scand J Gastroenterol. 1999;34:601–5.
27. Carmon E, Keidar A, Ravid A, Goldman G, Rabau M. The correlation between quality of life and functional outcome in ulcerative colitis patients after proctocolectomy ileal pouch anal anastomosis. Colorectal Dis. 2003;5:228–32.
28. Itzkowitz SH, Yio X. Inflammation and cancer iV. Colorectal cancer in inflammatory bowel disease: the role of inflammation. Am J Physiol Liver Physiol. 2004;287:G7–G17.
29. Breynaert C, Vermeire S, Rutgeerts P, Van Assche G. Dysplasia and colorectal cancer in inflammatory bowel disease: a result of inflammation or an intrinsic risk? Acta Gastroenterol Belg. 2008;71:367–72.
30. Shapiro BD, Lashner BA. Cancer biology in ulcerative colitis and potential use in endoscopic surveillance. Gastrointest Endosc Clin N Am. 1997;7:453–68.
31. Taylor BA, Wolff BG, Dozois RR, Kelly KA, Pemberton JH, Beart RW Jr. Ileal pouch-anal anastomosis for chronic ulcerative colitis and familial polyposis coli complicated by adenocarcinoma. Dis Colon Rectum. 1988;31:358–62.
32. Merchea A, Wolff BG, Dozois EJ, Abdelsattar ZM, Harmsen WS, Larson DW. Clinical features and oncologic outcomes in 77 patients with rectal cancer and ulcerative colitis: a single-institution experience. Dis Colon Rectum. 2012;55:881–5.

33. Gorfine SR, Harris MT, Bub DS, Bauer JJ. Restorative proctocolectomy for ulcerative colitis complicated by colorectal cancer. Dis Colon Rectum. 2004;47:1377–85.
34. Penna C, Tiret E, Daude F, Parc R. Results of ileal J-pouch-anal anastomosis in familial adenomatous polyposis complicated by rectal carcinoma. Dis Colon Rectum. 1994;37:157–60.
35. Radice E, Nelson H, Devine RM, Dozois RR, Nivatvongs S, Pemberton JH, Wolff BG, Fozard BJ, Ilstrup D. Ileal pouch- anal anastomosis in patients with colorectal cancer: long-term functional and oncologic outcomes. Dis Colon Rectum. 1998;41:11–7.
36. Remzi FH, Preen M. Rectal cancer and ulcerative colitis: does it change the therapeutic approach? Colorectal Dis. 2003;5:483–5.
37. Stelzner M, Fonkalsrud EW. The endorectal ileal pullthrough procedure in patients with ulcerative colitis and familial polyposis with carcinoma. Surg Gynecol Obstet. 1989;169:187–94.
38. Wiltz O, Hashmi HF, Schoetz DJ Jr, Roberts PL, Murray JJ, Coller JA, Veidenheimer MC. Carcinoma and the ileal pouch-anal anastomosis. Dis Colon Rectum. 1991;34:805–9.
39. Ziv Y, Fazio VW, Strong SA, Oakley JR, Milsom JW, Lavery IC. Ulcerative colitis and coexisting colorectal cancer: recurrence rate after restorative proctocolectomy. Ann Surg Oncol. 1994;1:512–5.
40. Ziv Y, Church JM, Oakley JR, McGannon E, Schroeder TK, Fazio VF. Results after restorative proctocolectomy and ileal pouch- anal anastomosis in patients with familial adenomatous polyposis and coexisting colorectal cancer. Br J Surg. 1996;83:1578–80.
41. Jung H, Beck-Bornholdt HP, Svoboda V, Alberti W, Herrmann T. Quantification of late complications after radiation therapy. Radiother Oncol. 2001;61:233–46.
42. Snelgrove R, Brown CJ, O'Connor BI, Huang H, Victor JC, Gryfe R, MacRae H, Cohen Z, McLeod RS. Proctocolectomy for colorectal cancer--is the ileal pouch anal anastomosis a safe alternative to permanent ileostomy? Int J Colorectal Dis. 2014;29(12):1485–91.
43. Heppell J, Weiland LH, Perrault J, Pemberton JH, Telander RL, Beart RW Jr. Fate of the rectal mucosa after rectal mucosectomy and ileoanal anastomosis. Dis Colon Rectum. 1983;26:768–71.
44. Setti-Carraro P, Ritchie JK, Wilkinson KH, Nicholls RJ, Hawley PR. The first 10 years' experience of restorative proctocolectomy for ulcerative colitis. Gut. 1994;35(8):1070–5.
45. Lewis WG, Sagar PM, Holdsworth PJ, Axon AT, Johnston D. Restorative proctocolectomy with end to end pouch-anal anastomosis in patients over the age of fifty. Gut. 1993;34:948–52.
46. Dayton MT, Larsen KR. Should older patients undergo ileal pouch-anal anastomosis? Am J Surg. 1996;172:444–7.
47. Reissman P, Teoh TA, Weiss EG, Nogueras JJ, Wexner SD. Functional outcome of the double stapled ileoanal reservoir in patients more than 60 years of age. Am Surg. 1996;62:178–83.
48. Bauer JJ, Gorfine SR, Gelernt IM, Harris MT, Kreel I. Restorative proctocolectomy in patients older than fifty years. Dis Colon Rectum. 1997;40:562–5.
49. Tan HT, Connolly AB, Morton D, Keighley MR. Results of restorative proctocolectomy in the elderly. Int J Colorectal Dis. 1997;12:319–22.
50. Takao Y, Gilliland R, Nogueras JJ, Weiss EG, Wexner SD. Is age relevant to functional outcome after restorative proctocolectomy for ulcerative colitis?: prospective assessment of 122 cases. Ann Surg. 1998;227:187–94.
51. Delaney CP, Fazio VW, Remzi FH, et al. Prospective, age- related analysis of surgical results, functional outcome, and quality of life after ileal pouch-anal anastomosis. Ann Surg. 2003;238:221–8.
52. Farouk R, Pemberton JH, Wolff BG, Dozois RR, Browning S, Larson D. Functional outcomes after ileal pouch-anal anastomosis for chronic ulcerative colitis. Ann Surg. 2000;231:919–26.
53. Ramage L, Qiu S, Georgiou P, et al. Functional outcomes following ileal pouch-anal anastomosis (IPAA) in older patients: a systematic review. Int J Colorectal Dis. 2016;31:481–92.
54. Hubbard RE, Story DA. Patient frailty: the elephant in the operating room. Anaesthesia. 2014;69:26–34.
55. Cohan JN, Bacchetti P, Varma MG, Finlayson E. Outcomes after ileoanal pouch surgery in frail and older adults. J Surg Res. 2015;198:327–33.

56. Ross H, Steele SR, Varma M, Dykes S, Cima R, Buie WD, Rafferty J, Standards Practice Task Force of the American Society of Colon and Rectal Surgeons. Practice parameters for the surgical treatment of ulcerative colitis. Dis Colon Rectum. 2014;57(1):5–22.
57. Long MD, Crandall WV, Leibowitz IH, Duffy L, del Rosario F, Kim SC, Integlia MJ, Berman J, Grunow J, Colletti RB, Schoen BT, Patel AS, Baron H, Israel E, Russell G, Ali S, Herfarth HH, Martin C, Kappelman MD. Prevalence and epidemiology of overweight and obesity in children with inflammatory bowel disease. Inflamm Bowel Dis. 2011;17:2162–8.
58. Efron JE, Uriburu JP, Wexner SD, Pikarsky A, Hamel C, Weiss EG, Nogueras JJ. Restorative proctocolectomy with ileal pouch anal anastomosis in obese patients. Obes Surg. 2001;11:246–51.
59. Kiran RP, Remzi FH, Fazio VW, Lavery IC, Church JM, Strong SA, Hull TL. Complications and functional results after ileoanal pouch formation in obese patients. J Gastrointest Surg. 2008;12:668–74.
60. Canedo JA, Pinto RA, McLemore EC, Rosen L, Wexner SD. Restorative proctectomy with ileal pouch–anal anastomosis in obese patients. Dis Colon Rectum. 2010;53:1030–4.
61. Klos CL, Safar B, Jamal N, et al. Obesity increases risk for pouch-related complications following restorative proctocolectomy with ileal pouch-anal anastomosis (IPAA). J Gastrointest Surg. 2014;18:573–9.
62. Ferrante M, D'Hoore A, Vermeire S, Declerck S, Noman M, Van Assche G, et al. Corticosteroids but not infliximab increase short-term postoperative infectious complications in patients with ulcerative colitis. Inflamm Bowel Dis. 2009;15:1062–70.
63. Mahadevan U, Loftus WJ Jr, Tremaine EV, Pemberton JH, Harmsen WS, Schleck CD, et al. Azathioprine or 6-mercaptopurine before colectomy for ulcerative colitis is not associated with increased postoperative complications. Inflamm Bowel Dis. 2002;8:311–6.
64. Mor IJ, Vogel JD, da Luz Moreira A, Shen B, Hammel J, Remzi FH. Infliximab in ulcerative colitis is associated with an increased risk of post- operative complications after restorative proctocolectomy. Dis Colon Rectum. 2008;51:1202–12077–10.
65. Selvasekar CR, Cima RR, Larson DW, Dozois EJ, Harrington JR, Harmsen WS, et al. Effect of infliximab on short-term complications in patients undergoing operation for chronic ulcerative colitis. J Am Coll Surg. 2007;204:956–96262–3.
66. Gainsbury ML, Chu DI, Howard LA, Coukos JA, Farraye FA, Stucchi AF, et al. Preoperative infliximab is not associated with an increased risk of short-term postoperative complications after restorative proctocolectomy and ileal pouch-anal anastomosis. J Gastrointest Surg. 2011;15:397–403.
67. Bregnbak D, Mortensen C, Bendtsen F. Infliximab and complications after colectomy in patients with ulcerative colitis. J Crohns Colitis. 2012;6:281–6.
68. Eshuis EJ, Al Saady RL, Stokkers PC, Ponsioen CY, Tanis PJ, Bemelman WA. Previous infliximab therapy and postoperative complications after proctocolectomy with ileum pouch anal anastomosis. J Crohns Colitis. 2013;7:142–9.
69. Pavlides M, Cleland J, Rahman M, et al. Outcomes after ileal pouch anal anastomosis in patients with primary sclerosing cholangitis. J Crohns Colitis. 2014;8:662–70.
70. Delaney CP, Remzi FH, Gramlich T, Dadvand B, Fazio VW. Equivalent function, quality of life and pouch survival rates after ileal-pouch anal anastomosis for indeterminate colitis and ulcerative colitis. Ann Surg. 2002;236:43–8.
71. Tekkis PP, Heriot AG, Smith O, Smith JJ, Windsor ACJ, Nicholls RJ. Long-term outcomes of restorative proctolectomy for Crohn's disease and indeterminate colitis. Colorectal Dis. 2005;7:218–23.
72. Antolovic D, Kienle P, Knaebel HP, Schmidt J, Gutt CN, Weitz J, et al. Totally laparoscopic versus conventional ileoanal pouch procedure– design of a single-centre, expertise based randomised controlled trial to compare the laparoscopic and conventional surgical approach in patients undergoing primary elective restorative proctocolectomy–LapConPouch- Trial. BMC Surg. 2006;6:13.

73. Tilney HS, Lovegrove RE, Heriot AG, Purkayastha S, Constantinides V, Nicholls RJ, et al. Comparison of short-term outcomes of laparoscopic vs open approaches to ileal pouch surgery. Int J Colorectal Dis. 2007;22:531–42.
74. Causey MW, Stoddard D, Johnson EK, et al. Laparoscopy impacts outcomes favourably following colectomy for ulcerative colitis: a critical analysis of the ACS-NSQIP database. Surg Endosc. 2013;27:603–9.
75. Ahmed AU, Keus F, Heikens JT, Bemelman WA, Berdah SV, Gooszen HG, et al. Open versus laparoscopic (assisted) ileo pouch anal anastomosis for ulcerative colitis and familial adenomatous polyposis. Cochrane Database Syst Rev. 2009;CD006267.
76. Dunker MS, Bemelman WA, Slors JF, van Duijvendijk P, Gouma DJ. Functional outcome, quality of life, body image, and cosmesis in patients after laparoscopic-assisted and conventional restorative proctocolectomy: a comparative study. Dis Colon Rectum. 2001;44:1800–7.
77. Fajardo AD, Dharmarajan S, George V, et al. Laparoscopic versus open 2-stage ileal pouch: laparoscopic approach allows for faster restoration of intestinal continuity. J Am Coll Surg. 2010;211:377–83.
78. Hull TL, Joyce MR, Geisler DP, Coffey JC. Adhesions after laparoscopic and open ileal pouch-anal anastomosis surgery for ulcerative colitis. Br J Surg. 2012;99:270–5.
79. Bartels SA, D'Hoore A, Cuesta MA, Bensdorp AJ, Lucas C, Bemelman WA. Significantly increased pregnancy rates after laparoscopic restorative proctocolectomy: a cross-sectional study. Ann Surg. 2012;256:1045–8.
80. Beyer-Berjot L, Maggiori L, Birnbaum D, Lefevre JH, Berdah S, Panis Y. A total laparoscopic approach reduces the infertility rate after ileal pouch-anal anastomosis: a 2-center study. Ann Surg. 2013;258(2):275–82.
81. Arbuthnot LW. The results of operative treatment of chronic constipation. BMJ. 1908;1:126–30.
82. Preston DM, Hawley PR, Lennard-Jones JE, et al. Results of colectomy for severe idiopathic constipation in women (Arbuthnot Lane's disease). Br J Surg. 1984;71(7):547–52.
83. Knowles CH, Scott M, Lunniss PJ. Outcome of colectomy for slow transit constipation. Ann Surg. 1999;230(5):627–38.
84. Mollen RM, Kuijpers HC, Claassen AT. Colectomy for slow-transit constipation: preoperative functional evaluation is important but not a guarantee for a successful outcome. Dis Colon Rectum. 2001;44(4):577–80.
85. Gladman MA, Scott SM, Lunniss PJ, et al. Systematic review of surgical options for idiopathic megarectum and megacolon. Ann Surg. 2005;241:562–74.
86. Nicholls RJ, Kamm MA. Proctocolectomy with restorative ileoanal reservoir for severe idiopathic constipation. Report of two cases. Dis Colon Rectum. 1988;31(12):968–9.
87. Hosie KB, Kmiot WA, Keighley MR. Constipation: another indication for restorative proctocolectomy. Br J Surg. 1990;77:801–2.
88. Stewart J, Kumar D, Keighley MR. Results of anal or low rectal anastomosis and pouch construction for megarectum and megacolon. Br J Surg. 1994;81:1051–3.
89. Kalbassi MR, Winter DC, Deasy JM. Quality-of-life assessment of patients after ileal pouch–anal anastomosis for slow-transit constipation with rectal inertia. Dis Colon Rectum. 2003;46:1508–12.

# Chapter 3
# Pouch Configuration

**Antonino Spinelli and Marco Ettore Allaix**

**Abstract** Restorative proctocolectomy with ileal pouch-anal anastomosis (IPAA) is the standard of care for the surgical treatment of patients with ulcerative colitis (UC). The J-pouch is the configuration of choice in patients undergoing restorative proctocolectomy for UC. Hand-sewn and stapled IPAA have a similar safety profile, while functional outcomes are better in patients with stapled pouch. The indications for hand-sewn and stapled pouch in patients with rectal dysplasia or cancer are under evaluation.

**Keywords** Ulcerative colitis · Pouch · Hand-sewn · Stapled · Functional outcomes

## 3.1 Introduction

Restorative proctocolectomy with ileal pouch-anal anastomosis (IPAA) is the surgical procedure of choice for the treatment of chronic ulcerative colitis (UC) [1], with durable functional outcomes and good quality of life in most UC patients even 30 years after surgery [2].

Since 1978, several ileal reservoirs have been conceived. The hand-sewn three-limb S-pouch [3] was soon replaced by the hand-sewn J-pouch [4] and W-pouch [5], that were associated with better functional outcomes than the S-pouch [6]. The development of the staplers in the early 1980s has raised several questions about the best method to construct the IPAA and the outcomes in patients with a stapled pouch [7].

A. Spinelli (✉)
Humanitas University, Department of Biomedical Sciences, Rozzano, Milano, Italy

Humanitas Clinical and Research Center, Division of Colon and Rectal Surgery, Rozzano, Milano, Italy
e-mail: antonino.spinelli@hunimed.eu

M. E. Allaix
Department of Surgical Sciences, University of Torino, Torino, Italy

 
J. Warusavitarne, Z. Perry-Woodford (eds.), *The Ileoanal Pouch*,
https://doi.org/10.1007/978-3-319-94385-5_3

The aims of this chapter are to critically compare the outcomes of different pouch designs, discuss the oncologic outcomes in patients undergoing hand-sewn or stapled IPAA for UC associated with dysplasia or cancer, and to report the technique in our institution.

## 3.2 The Pouch: S-, J- or W?

The configurations include J-, S- and W- pouches. As recently stated with a high level of evidence by the European Crohn's and Colitis Organisation (ECCO), "the J-pouch is the standard of care due to its simplicity to construct and good long-term function outcome" [8].

The first pouch described in 1978 was the three-limb S pouch that used the terminal 30 cm of the small bowel; a 25- cm segment was opened on the antimesenteric aspect and folded three times, while the terminal 5-cm segment acted as a conduit [3].

A few years later, Utsunomiya et al. [4] proposed a two-limb J pouch, while Nicholls described a four-limb W pouch aiming to overcome the need for pouch intubation to facilitate defecation [5].

### *3.2.1 The Evidence*

These three pouch configurations have similar morbidity rates. A meta-analysis of short-term and long-term outcomes of J-, W- and S-ileal reservoirs for restorative proctocolectomy including 1519 patients [6] found no significant differences in IPAA leak rates, strictures and mortality. Pelvic sepsis occurred in 15% of J pouch patients, 7% of W pouch patients and 19.6% of S pouch patients. Pouchitis occurred in 18% of J pouch patients, in 13% of W pouch patients and 15.5% of S pouch patients. Pouch failure was observed in 7.3%, 0% and 6.3% of patients, respectively.

Regarding functional outcomes, daily stool frequency, the need for anti-diarrheal medication and the use of protective pads are significantly greater after a J reservoir than W or S reservoir, while there are no significant differences between W and S reservoir. A higher number of bowel movements is the consequence of a small volume pouch and tends to reduce over the years. The J pouch configuration is associated with significantly lower rates of evacuation issues requiring anal intubation than the W and S pouch (1.8% vs. 20% vs. 29.6%, respectively). The three configurations are similar in terms of incontinence and resting pressure or peak squeeze pressure, suggesting that compliance of the ileal pouch and intact anal sphincter physiology are more important than the pouch configuration in determining the outcomes.

To date, a few studies have investigated the quality of life in patients undergoing IPAA for UC and data concerning the pouch configuration are very limited. For instance, Wade et al. [9] have retrospectively reviewed 49 patients who had IPAA with J pouch (N = 30) or W pouch (N = 19). A questionnaire including 10 questions about quality of life was mailed to all patients and a telephone survey was performed when the patient did not return the questionnaire. General health status, mental status, activity restrictions, urgency, seepage during the day and at night, protective use during the day and at night were similar. These results, while not randomized, comparing J and W pouch, support the J pouch as the configuration of choice in patients undergoing restorative proctocolectomy for UC.

## 3.3 IPAA: Hand-Sewn or Stapled?

The introduction of stapling devices in the early 1980s has led to different techniques described for IPAA construction: rectal stump mucosectomy followed by hand-sewn pouch and stapled pouch with preservation of the rectal mucosa. The hand-sewn IPAA has the advantage of completely removing the potentially diseased or inflamed rectal mucosa, while the main drawbacks are longer operative time, greater manipulation of the anal canal with higher risks of postoperative anal dysfunction. In addition, the excision of the mucosa of the anal transition zone that is involved in maintaining the anorectal inhibitory reflex, plays a role in decreasing the ability to discriminate between gas and stool [10–19].

Many studies have compared hand-sewn and stapled IPAA following proctocolectomy. In 2006, Lovegrove et al. [20] have included in a meta-analysis 21 comparative studies (6 randomized controlled trials, 5 prospective studies, 10 retrospective studies), consisting of 4183 patients: 2699 underwent hand-sewn and 1484 stapled IPAA between 1983 and 2000. A J pouch was created in 3184 patients (80.1%), while a S-pouch or a W-pouch was constructed in 743 (18.7%) and 49 (1.2%) patients, respectively. Mean follow-up was 26.8 months in the hand-sewn group and 19.6 months in the stapled group. There were no significant differences in the rates of overall postoperative morbidity, anastomotic leak, pelvic sepsis, anastomotic stricture, pouch-related fistula, small bowel obstruction, wound infection, pouchitis, ileal pouch failure and mortality between the two groups. The analysis of functional outcomes showed that the two techniques are similar in stool frequency per 24 h, defecation at night, use of antidiarrheal medications and seepage during daytime. Patients undergoing hand-sewn IPAA experienced incontinence of liquid stool more often than patients treated with stapled IPAA. Nocturnal seepage and the use of pads overnight were both more common after hand-sewn IPAA. These poorer outcomes are associated with a significant decrease in both resting and squeeze pressure among hand-sewn patients. Lastly, there are no significant differences in quality of life and sexual dysfunctions in both male and female patients after hand-sewn or stapled IPAA.

A few years later, Kirat et al. [21] performed a retrospective review of 3109 patients undergoing a primary IPAA. A total of 474 patients had a hand-sewn IPAA and 2635 a stapled IPAA. The two groups of patients were similar, except for a higher number of patients with defunctioning stoma in the hand-sewn group and more J-pouches in the stapled group. With a mean follow-up of 7.1 years, the authors found that patients with hand-sewn IPAA had more anastomotic strictures, septic complications, postoperative small bowel obstruction and failure of the pouch. These conflicting results compared to the Lovegrove's metanalysis findings might be related to the number of patients included in the studies, the definition of the complications, the use of protective stoma and the length of follow-up. The analysis of functional outcomes showed that incontinence, seepage, pad usage, dietary, social and work restrictions were more frequent in patients who had a hand-sewn IPAA. As a consequence, these patients reported poorer quality of life, health and lower happiness with the operation than patients who had a stapled IPAA.

Despite hand-sewn and stapled IPAA having similar anastomotic leak rates, there is some evidence showing better functional outcomes and lower pouch failure rates after a leak with a stapled IPAA. For instance, Lian et al. [22] evaluated 175 patients with anastomotic leak (34 hand-sewn and 141 stapled IPAA). Patients undergoing hand-sewn IPAA were younger, received less steroids preoperatively, had more proximal diversion and S-pouches than patients with stapled IPAA. IPAA failure rate was 35% among the hand-sewn patients and 12% among the stapled patients. Leak after hand-sewn IPAA was an independent risk factor of IPAA failure and was associated with higher incontinence rate at 5 years after surgery and higher nocturnal seepage rate at long-term follow-up.

Patients with UC are at higher risk of developing colorectal cancer. The indications for hand-sewn or stapled IPAA in patients with high-grade dysplasia or rectal cancer are unclear. While mucosectomy is proposed as procedure of choice based on the potential risk of cancer development within the residual rectal mucosa in case of stapled IPAA [23], there are several reports showing cancer occurrence even in patients undergoing hand-sewn IPAA [24–28], likely secondary to incomplete removal of the inflamed rectal mucosa. Al-Sukhni et al. c published a large series of patients with UC and colorectal dysplasia or cancer, aiming to assess the rate of dysplasia or cancer at IPAA. A total of 81 patients were included: 59 with stapled IPAA and 22 with ghand-sewn IPAA. With a median follow-up of 76.1 months, stapled IPAA did not appear to lead to worse oncologic outcomes than mucosectomy and handsewn IPAA. However, further large studies with long follow-up are needed to better answer the question about the best pouch construction in these subgroup of patients.

## 3.4 Our Technique

It is our practice to perform a J-pouch with a double stapled IPAA. In order to create a tension-free anastomosis, the small bowel mesentery should be sufficiently mobilized up to the horizontal part of the duodenum, to allow the J-pouch to reach the level of the levator muscles [30].

The pouch is constructed using the most dependent loop of distal bowel. The ileum is folded into two portions of about 15 cm. An enterotomy of about 1.5 cm is performed longitudinally at the apex of the two folded ileal segments. A side-to-side anastomosis of the two portions of distal ileum is created, usually by 2 fires of a linear stapler, 100 mm. The blind loop of the J-pouch is sealed by linear stapler and oversewn by running suture and solidarized to the afferent limb in order to prevent dilation. The ileal pouch is then flushed with saline to confirm the patency of the suture and the stapled lines are checked for hemostasis. Interrupted 4/0 stitches are placed in case of bleeding along the suture lines. Afterwards, a 0-polypropylene purse string is made at the margin of the enterotomy. A 31 mm anvil is placed at the apex of the pouch and a standard double stapled end-to-end anastomosis is created with a circular stapler, advanced through the anus. Before the staple firing, the pouch should be adequately oriented in order to avoid twisting of the mesentery. In female patients, attention must be payed to avoid the inclusion of the posterior wall of the vagina within the staple line. The doughnuts are checked for completeness.

More recently, we started to perform a double purse string anastomosis after the introduction, in our practice, of transanal proctectomy (TAMIS pouch) and single-port abdominal laparoscopic surgery.

## References


1. Michelassi F, Lee J, Rubin M, Fichera A, Kasza K, Karrison T, Hurst RD. Long-term functional results after ileal pouch anal restorative proctocolectomy for ulcerative colitis: a prospective observational study. Ann Surg. 2003;238(3):433–41; discussion 442-5.
2. Lightner AL, Mathis KL, Dozois EJ, Hahnsloser D, Loftus EV Jr, Raffals LE, Pemberton JH. Results at up to 30 years after ileal pouch-anal anastomosis for chronic ulcerative colitis. Inflamm Bowel Dis. 2017; https://doi.org/10.1097/MIB.0000000000001061. [Epub ahead of print].
3. Parks AG, Nicholls RJ. Proctocolectomy without ileostomy for ulcerative colitis. BMJ. 1978;2:85–8.
4. Utsunomiya J, Iwama T, Imajo M, Matsuo S, Sawai S, Yaegashi K, Hirayama R. Total colectomy, mucosal proctectomy, and ileoanal anastomosis. Dis Colon Rectum. 1980;23:459–66.
5. Nicholls RJ. Restorative proctocolectomy with ileal reservoir: indications and results. Schweiz Med Wochenschr. 1990;120:485–8.
6. Lovegrove RE, Heriot AG, Constantinides V, Tilney HS, Darzi AW, Fazio VW, Nicholls RJ, Tekkis PP. Meta-analysis of short-term and long-term outcomes of J, W and S ileal reservoirs for restorative proctocolectomy. Colorectal Dis. 2007;9(4):310–20.
7. Bach SP, Mortensen NJM. Revolution and evolution: 30 years of ileoanal pouch surgery. Inflamm Bowel Dis. 2006;12:131–45.
8. Øresland T, Bemelman WA, Sampietro GM, Spinelli A, Windsor A, Ferrante M, Marteau P, Zmora O, Kotze PG, Espin-Basany E, Tiret E, Sica G, Panis Y, Faerden AE, Biancone L, Angriman I, Serclova Z, de Buck van Overstraeten A, Gionchetti P, Stassen L, Warusavitarne J, Adamina M, Dignass A, Eliakim R, Magro F, D'Hoore A, European Crohn's and Colitis Organisation (ECCO). European evidence based consensus on surgery for ulcerative colitis. J Crohns Colitis. 2015;9(1):4–25.
9. Wade AD, Mathiason MA, Brekke EF, Kothari SN. Quality of life after ileoanal pouch: a comparison of J ans W puoches. J Gastrointest Surg. 2009;13:1260–5.
10. Pemberton JH, Kelly KA, Beart RW Jr, Dozois RR, Wolff BG, Ilstrup DM. Ileal pouch-anal anastomosis for chronic ulcerative colitis. Long-term results. Ann Surg. 1987;206:504–13.

11. Wexner SD, Jensen L, Rothenberger DA, Wong WD, Goldberg SM. Long-term functional analysis of the ileoanal reservoir. Dis Colon Rectum. 1989;32:275–81.
12. Choen S, Tsunoda A, Nicholls RJ. Prospective randomized trial comparing anal function after hand sewn ileoanal anastomosis with mucosectomy versus stapled ileoanal anastomosis without mucosectomy in restorative proctocolectomy. Br J Surg. 1991;78:430–4.
13. Tuckson W, Lavery I, Fazio V, Oakley J, Church J, Milsom J. Manometric and functional comparison of ileal pouch anal anastomosis with and without anal manipulation. Am J Surg. 1991;161:90–5.
14. Johnston D, Holdsworth PJ, Nasmyth DG, et al. Preservation of the entire anal canal in conservative proctocolectomy for ulcerative colitis: a pilot study comparing end-to-end ileo-anal anastomosis without mucosal resection with mucosal proctectomy and endo-anal anastomosis. Br J Surg. 1987;74:940–4.
15. Holdsworth PJ, Johnston D. Anal sensation after restorative proctocolectomy for ulcerative colitis. Br J Surg. 1988;75:993–6.
16. Heald RJ, Allen DR. Stapled ileo-anal anastomosis: a technique to avoid mucosal proctectomy in the ileal pouch operation. Br J Surg. 1986;73:571–2.
17. Sagar PM, Holdsworth PJ, Johnston D. Correlation between laboratory findings and clinical outcome after restorative proctocolectomy: serial studies in 20 patients with end-to-end pouch-anal anastomosis. Br J Surg. 1991;78:67–70.
18. Sugerman HJ, Newsome HH. Stapled ileoanal anastomosis without a temporary ileostomy. Am J Surg. 1994;167:58–65.
19. Reilly WT, Pemberton JH, Wolff BG, et al. Randomized prospective trial comparing ileal pouch-anal anastomosis performed by excising the anal mucosa to ileal pouch-anal anastomosis performed by preserving the anal mucosa. Ann Surg. 1997;225:666–76.
20. Lovegrove RE, Constantinides VA, Heriot AG, Athanasiou T, Darzi A, Remzi FH, Nicholls RJ, Fazio VW, Tekkis PP. A comparison of hand-sewn versus stapled ileal pouch anal anastomosis (IPAA) following proctocolectomy: a meta-analysis of 4183 patients. Ann Surg. 2006;244(1):18–26.
21. Kirat HT, Remzi FH, Kiran RP, Fazio VW. Comparison of outcomes after hand-sewn versus staples ileal piuch-anal anastomosis in 3109 patients. Surgery. 2009;146:723–30.
22. Lian L, Kiran RP, Remzi FH, Lavery IC, Fazio VW. Outcomes for patients developing anastomotic leak after ileal pouch-anal anastomosis: does a handsewn vs. stapled anastomosis matter? Dis Colon Rectum. 2009;52:387–93.
23. Remzi FH, Preen M. Rectal cancer and ulcerative colitis: does it change the therapeutic approach? Colorectal Dis. 2003;5:483–5.
24. Chambers WM, McC Mortensen NJ. Should ileal pouch-anal anastomosis include mucosectomy? Colorectal Dis. 2007;9:384–92.
25. Vento P, Lepisto A, Karkkainen P, Ristimaki A, Haglund C, Jarvinen HJ. Risk of cancer in patients with chronic pouchitis after restorative proctocolectomy for ulcerative colitis. Colorectal Dis. 2011;13(1):58–66.
26. Branco BC, Sachar DB, Heimann TM, Sarpel U, Harpaz N, Greenstein AJ. Adenocarcinoma following ileal pouch-anal anastomosis for ulcerative colitis: review of 26 cases. Inflamm Bowel Dis. 2009;15:295–9.
27. Ault GT, Nunoo-Mensah JW, Johnson L, Vukasin P, Kaiser A, Beart RW Jr. Adenocarcinoma arising in the middle of ileoanal pouches: report of five cases. Dis Colon Rectum. 2009;52:538–41.
28. Panier-Suffat L, Marracino M, Resegotti A, Astegiano M, Giustetto A, Garino M, Pellicano R, Fronda G. Anal transitional zone adenocarcinoma following restorative proctocolectomy for ulcerative colitis: case report and review of literature. Acta Gastroenterol Belg. 2009;72:441–3.
29. Al-Sukhni W, McLeod RS, MacRae H, O'Connor B, Huang H, Cohen Z. Oncologic outcome in patients with ulcerative colitis associated with dysplasia or cancer who underwent stapled or handsewn ileal pouch-anal anastomosis. Dis Colon Rectum. 2010;53:1495–500.
30. Leo CA, Samaranayake S, Perry-Woodford ZL, Vitone L, Faiz O, Hodgkinson JD, Shaikh I, Warusavitarne J. Initial experience of restorative proctocolectomy for ulcerative colitis by transanal total mesorectal rectal excision and single-incision abdominal laparoscopic surgery. Colorectal Dis. 2016;18(12):1162–6.

# Chapter 4
# Pouch Lengthening Techniques

**Elaine Burns and Robin Phillips**

**Abstract** One concern in pouch surgery is creating an ileal pouch-anal anastomosis (IPAA) that is as tension-free as possible. Another is avoiding the embarrassing scenario of a pouch in one hand and the anus in the other with insufficient length to bring the two together. The key to all this involves early assessment of potential length in order to identify those few cases in time where there may be difficulty and the right strategy may obviate that difficulty. This chapter seeks to outline the techniques (Fig. 4.1) available to the surgeon to allow a tension free anastomosis and suggests possible lengthening measures in those particularly challenging cases.

**Keywords** Pouch length · Vascular anatomy · Vascular anatomy of the ileum

The principle steps involve thorough mobilisation of the small bowel mesentery, horizontal front and back peritoneal incisions in the small bowel mesentery, pouch design, pouch orientation, and an understanding of how the vascular anatomy can be used to advantage.

One should bear in mind that complete lack of tension may not always be a good thing. With time or too much length, the pouch may start to kink at the pouch-anal anastomosis, leading to the pouch dislocating from on top of the anus and falling sideways, thereby obstructing defaecation and requiring the need to empty with a Medena catheter, as was seen in 50% of initial S-pouch designs over time. This is probably because the S-pouch design does indeed supply additional length, useful in some cases, critically useful in a minority with a very short mesentery, but a potential Achilles' heel when length is sufficient and too much length a disadvantage.

It is therefore important to assess the reach of the small bowel deep into the pelvis at the outset of the operation. The potential future pouch (at this time represented by the most dependent distal loop of ileum and situated around 20 cm upstream of

E. Burns · R. Phillips (✉)
St. Mark's Hospital, Harrow, UK

Imperial College, London, UK
e-mail: e.burns@imperial.ac.uk; robin.phillips@nhs.net

 
J. Warusavitarne, Z. Perry-Woodford (eds.), *The Ileoanal Pouch*,
https://doi.org/10.1007/978-3-319-94385-5_4

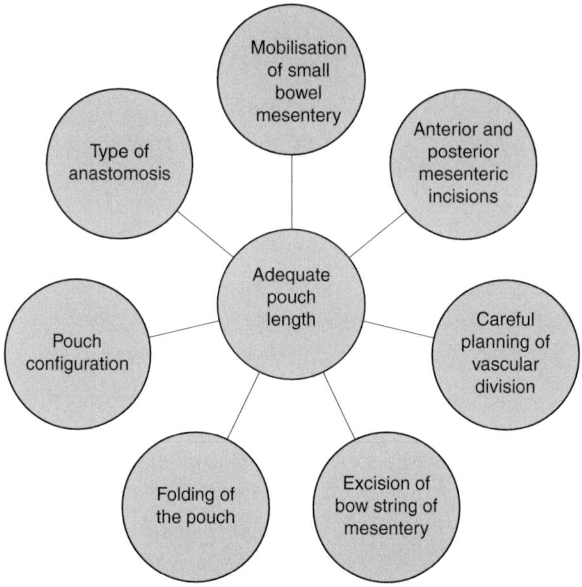


**Fig. 4.1** Key steps to gaining sufficient length

**Table 4.1** Reach of pouch and consequent percentage of likely tension free anastomosis

| Distance from the inferior margin of symphysis pubis | Percentage of pouches to dentate line without tension |
|---|---|
| 6 cm | 100 |
| 4 cm | 55 |
| 2 cm | 33 |

Smith et al. [11]

the ileocaecal valve) should reach beyond the inferior border of the pubic symphysis. The surgeon should allow for a greater reach than the symphysis alone as the distance to the pubic symphysis is less than the distance to the dentate line. Smith and colleagues assessed the reach beyond the lower border of the pubic symphysis required to achieve what the authors designated a tension-free pouch-anal anastomosis [11]. They assessed 12 cadaver cases and measured the reach to the dentate line relative to the pubic symphysis. As outlined in Table 4.1, a distance of 6 cm below the pubic symphysis achieved a tension free anastomosis in 100% of cases.

In some cases, attaining the necessary pouch length can be challenging and a range of manoeuvres are required to achieve sufficient length. The small bowel mesentery should be mobilised in its entirety. The peritoneum of the small bowel mesentery can be incised both anteriorly and posteriorly with careful preservation of the vasculature. Excision of any 'bowstring' of avascular mesentery can gain valuable length. Beyond these measures, careful consideration of the vascular supply to the pouch is required (Fig. 4.1).

## 4.1 Mobilisation of Small Bowel Mesentery

Mobilisation of the entire small bowel mesentery from the duodenum and ligament of Treitz is essential to maximise small bowel length. The second and third part of duodenum should be exposed. Mobilisation of the root of the SMA gained 0.5–1 cm in length in a cadaveric study in 6/13 cases [4]. Following this manoeuvre, sufficient length may be obtained by division of smaller vascular arcades and thickened peritoneum.

## 4.2 Anterior and Posterior Mesenteric Incisions

The peritoneum of the small bowel mesentery may be incised both anteriorly and posteriorly in a stepladder fashion [2, 8]. Such incisions are thought to gain approximately 1 cm in length in those with normal peritoneum and 2 cm in those patients with thickened mesentery [3]. Khurrum Baig and colleagues suggested this technique could gain, in fact, 4–8 cm in length when combined with division of the ileocolic artery and associated fat with no increase in complications [2]. The division of the smaller vascular arcades causing tension with the creation of a mesenteric window can also confer an extra 2–5 cm in length, but should be done with great care and vascularity tested before division by the use of bulldog clips [3].

## 4.3 Careful Planning of Vascular Division

If these measures do not achieve the desired mobility of the pouch careful consideration should be given to the vascular supply of the pouch. The available length of the small bowel mesentery and the terminal ileal vascular anatomy should be assessed at an early stage to allow careful planning of the pouch vasculature to maximise pouch length.

The vascular supply to the terminal ileum receives contributions from the superior mesenteric artery via the terminal branch and the ileocolic artery via the caecal and the ileal branches (Fig. 4.2). The right colic artery and the middle colic artery via the marginal vascular arcade also contribute in some patients.

The standard approach to vascular division is to ligate the right colic and ileocolic flush with the SMA and rely on the SMA to supply the pouch. The window of peritoneum between the ileocolic vessels and the continuing superior mesenteric vessels act as a bow-string, restricting pouch advancement and needing excision. However, at the outset of the operation it is important to assess whether ileocolic artery or the continuing superior mesenteric vessel resists the pelvic descent of the pouch. This allows planning of the vascular supply of the pouch.

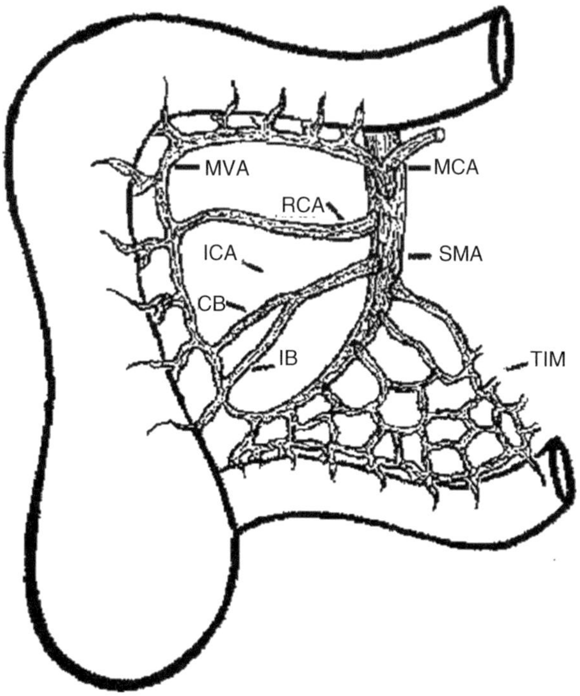


**Fig. 4.2** Anatomy to the terminal ileum and right colon. MCA middle colic artery, RCA right colic artery, ICA ileocolic artery, CB caecal branch, IB ileal branch, SMA superior mesenteric branch, MVA marginal vascular arcade, TIM terminal ileal mesentery. (Reproduced with permission from Goes et al. [6])

Smith and colleagues in a cadaver study showed that the longest branch of the SMA is up to 8 cm longer than the ileocaecal artery [11]. In the event that such a ligation would not allow sufficient length, other vascular configurations have been suggested.

In an angiographic cadaver study, the terminal branch of the ileocolic artery and SMA formed an anastomotic loop in all 13 cases allowing division of either vessel to gain length [4]. Such vascular divisions provided a gain of 5 cm in 80% of the 13 cases studied in this cadaveric experiment. In 23% of cases, in the cadaveric study, the recurrent ileal branch was the only blood supply to the terminal ileum [4].

If sufficient length is not possible with this manoeuvre, in some circumstances, the marginal vascular arcade of the right colon can act as the blood supply to the ileal pouch [6]. But in doing this, a close colonic dissection is necessary and associated lymph nodes are not removed, so the technique should not be used when there is a realistic prospect of cancer in the caecum or ascending colon. Division of the ileocolic artery or the superior mesenteric artery (SMA) with preservation of the marginal vascular arcade of the right colon are both possibilities. Goes and colleagues in a further cadaveric study found that division of the ileocaecal and right colonic arteries allowed greatest mobilisation with a gain of 7.5 cm [7]. In these studies, division of the distal SMA, ileocaecal artery and right colic vessels achieved the most gain in mesenteric length. Such a technique relies on flow from the marginal vascular artery from the middle colic distally and the ileal branches of the SMA distally. Goes and colleagues suggested that such vascular division could achieve an additional mesenteric length of 36% (9.1 cm) [6]. In a cadaver study of six patients, Goes and colleagues assessed the additional length gained from the division/preservation of the three main vessels. They found that reliance on the marginal vascular arcade form the middle colic artery allowed an addition 3.6 cm in length [7]. Such an approach will depend on which vessels were divided during any prior colectomy.

Araki and colleagues investigated the impact of such techniques on early complications [1]. They included patients with inflammatory and non-inflammatory indications for pouch surgery and found no differences in outcome according to which vessels were divided at the time of formation of their pouch. The cohort was divided into those patients in whom the superior mesenteric artery, ileocolic artery and marginal vascular arcades were divided or preserved. In this study sufficient length was considered as the ability to distract a fixed point on ileum, 20 cm from the ileocaecal valve, to 2 cm beyond the symphysis pubis. This study only included those patients undergoing a primary open restorative proctocolectomy. Minimally invasive procedures were not included. Over a 66 month period, 220 patients who underwent a pouch procedure were included. Overall 55% of patients needed a lengthening technique. Of these, three vessels (ICA, SMA, MVA) were preserved in 34.5% of the patients with 2 vessels preserved in 52% of the patients. The SMA was most commonly sacrificed in this group. The overall defunctioning ileostomy rate was 47% of procedures. The choice of lengthening technique did not affect the rate of complications following the procedure. It appears that, given reasonable vascularisation of the pouch, gaining adequate length is more important than the technique used to gain this adequate length. By carefully detailing the vascular anatomy early in the operation, the authors were able to anastomose 220 out of 221 patients.

Martel and colleagues compared outcome in 21 patients who had a high division of the superior mesenteric pedicle with 44 patients in whom this was preserved in a retrospective study [10]. High division involved clamping the superior mesenteric pedicle at the level of the last division of the jejunal vessel. This relied on vascularization of the ileum by the ileocolic pedicle. This manoeuvre gained 5–7 cm in additional length in these 21 patients. There were no differences in complication rates between the two groups though the overall numbers were small. Figure 4.3 shows the arterial supply to the pouch is reliant on the marginal artery.

## 4.4 Excision of Bow String of Mesentery

It is important to dissect out the bow string of mesentery that remains following division of the vessel [1] (Fig. 4.4). This will gain extra valuable length. It may also be necessary carefully to divide occasional arcade vessels between vasa recta and terminal branch of the SMA having previously tested with bulldog clips.

It may be necessary to preserve the marginal artery from the middle colic to ensure sufficient length.

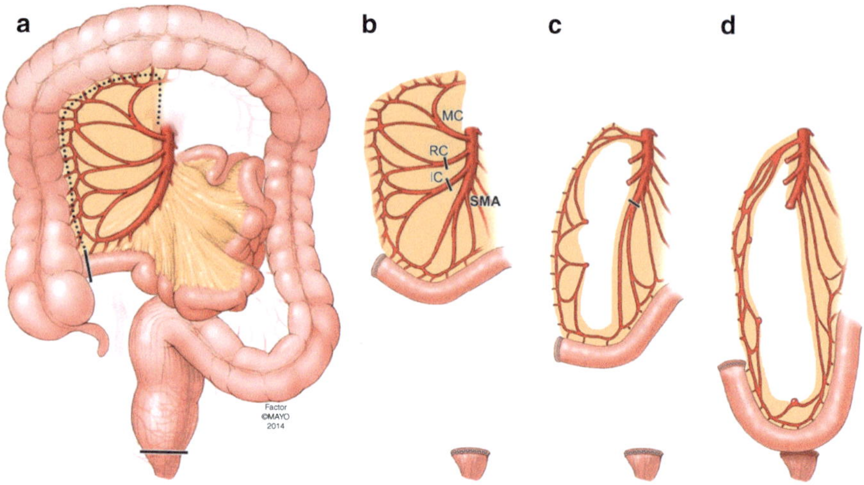


**Fig. 4.3** Advanced ileal pouch-anal anastomosis (IPAA) reconstruction. Overview strategy showing the correct line of transection during the colectomy (**a**) to preserve the critical mesenteric vessels including the superior mesenteric artery (SMA), ileocolic artery (IC), right colic artery (RC), and middle colic artery (MC). Ligation of the RC and IC (**b**) preserves blood flow from the preserved MC via the right marginal arteries and provides additional length in pouch reach. (**c**, **d**) Ligation of the distal SMA provides the final and most significant gain in length for the construction of a tension-free IPAA with critical blood supply from the MC. (Reproduced with permission from Chu et al. [5])

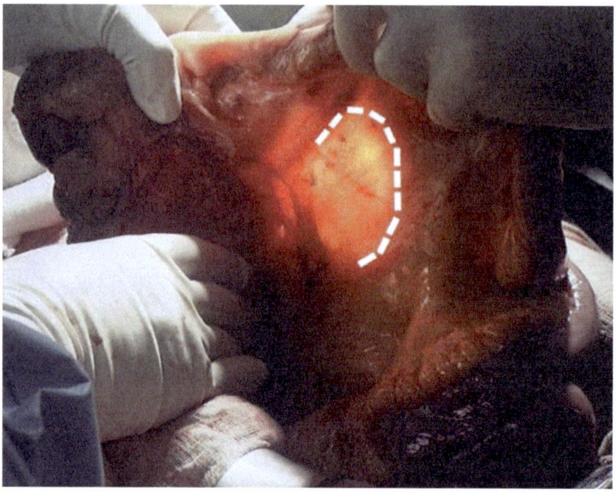

**Fig. 4.4** Excision of bowstring. Bowstring of mesentery demarcated by dotted line. (Adapted from http://www.stmarksacademicinstitute.org.uk/resources/gaining-length-in-pouch-surgery/)

## 4.5 Further Techniques to Increase Length

### *4.5.1 Vary the Apex of the Pouch*

It may be useful to vary the apex of the pouch according to the distance from the ileocaecal valve with a more proximal apex allowing less tension during pelvic descent [9].

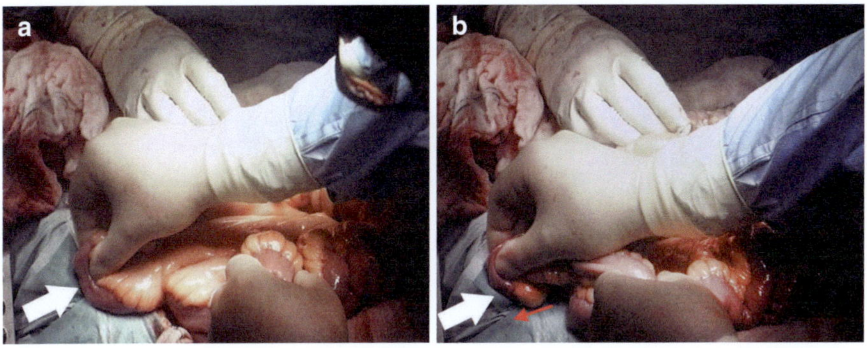


**Fig. 4.5** Change in length with pouch folding. (**a**) Pouch folded posteriorly. White arrow represents caudal reach of pouch. (**b**) Pouch folded anteriorly. White arrow represents caudal reach of pouch and red arrow represents additional length gained. (Adapted from http://www.stmarksacademicinstitute.org.uk/resources/gaining-length-in-pouch-surgery/)

### *4.5.2 Folding of the Pouch*

Folding of the pouch anteriorly allows an extra gain of potentially 1–2 cm in length. If the mesentery lies anteriorly the pouch will neatly follow the sacral hollow but the reach at the tip is slightly reduced. Placing the pouch anteriorly and the mesentery posteriorly gains length (Fig. 4.5).

## 4.6 Pouch Configuration

An S-shaped pouch does reach further than a J-shaped pouch. On a cadaver study, Cherqui and colleagues found that an S shaped pouch allowed a mean increase in length of 0.68 cm [4]. Earlier work by Smith et al. suggested that an S-shaped pouch reached 2 cm caudally when compared with a J-shaped pouch [11]. The S-shaped pouch can be associated with evacuatory difficulties. This is probably when the additional length is unnecessary, leading to a floppy pouch that can dislocate off the top of the pouch, obstructing defaecation. But in those cases where one is struggling to gain adequate reach of the pouch, it seems unlikely that such pouch dislocation would arise.

## 4.7 Type of Anastomosis

A hand sewn anastomosis requires more length than a stapled anastomosis. The question as to whether in difficult circumstances permitting an additional rectal cuff in order to take advantage of this point would be acceptable depends on the underlying pathology but in these authors' views might in exceptional circumstances be adopted.

Sufficient pelvic reach of the pouch is a necessary component of pouch surgery. This chapter has described a series of manouevres that taken together should allow the surgeon safely to perform an ileal pouch-anal anastomosis. These steps require careful thought with early consideration of the vasculature of the pouch as well as which vessels represent the limiting factor. Each step may contribute a small increase in length but taken together they will usually allow a successful outcome.

Reference video http://www.stmarksacademicinstitute.org.uk/resources/gaining-length-in-pouch-surgery/

## References

1. Araki T, et al. The effect on morbidity of mesentery lengthening techniques and the use of a covering stoma after Ileoanal pouch surgery. Dis Colon Rectum. 2006;49:621–8.
2. Baig MK, et al. Lengthening of small bowel mesentery: stepladder incision technique. Am J Surg. 2006;191:715–7.
3. Burnstein MJ, Schoetz DJ Jr, Coller JA, Veidenheimer MC. Technique of mesenteric lengthening in ileal reservoir-anal anastomosis. Dis Colon Rectum. 1987;30:863–6.
4. Cherqui D, Valleur P, Perniceni T, Hautefeuille P. Inferior reach of ileal reservoir in ileoanal anastomosis. Experimental anatomic and angiographic study. Dis Colon Rectum. 1987;30:365–71.
5. Chu DI, et al. Strategy for the difficult-to-reach ileal pouch-anal anastomosis: technical steps of an in vivo application of a mesenteric-lengthening technique. Tech Coloproctolo. 2015;19:705–9.
6. Goes RN, Nguyen P, Huang D, Beart RW Jr. Lengthening of the mesentery using the marginal vascular arcade of the right colon as the blood supply to the ileal pouch. Dis Colon Rectum. 1995;38:893–5.
7. Goes RN, Coy CS, Amaral CA, Fagundes JJ, Medeiros RR. Superior mesenteric artery syndrome as a complication of ileal pouch-anal anastomosis. Report of a case. Dis Colon Rectum. 1995;38:543–4.
8. Levine LA. Stepladder incision technique for lengthening of bowel mesentry. J Urol. 1992;148:351–2.
9. Ma RWL, Gold DM. Ileoanal pouch: short mesentery? Lengthen the pouch. Ann R Coll Surg Engl. 2011;93:488–9.
10. Martel P, et al. Mesenteric lengthening in ileoanal pouch anastomosis for ulcerative colitis: is high division of the superior mesenteric pedicle a safe procedure? Dis Colon Rectum. 1998;41:862–6.
11. Smith L, Friend WG, Medwell SJ. The superior mesenteric artery: the critical factor in the pouch pull-through procedure. Dis Colon Rectum. 1984;27:741–4.

# Chapter 5
# Minimally Invasive Pouch Surgery: Tips and Tricks

**Nicola Hodges and Janindra Warusavitarne**

**Abstract** Minimally invasive surgery for ileoanal pouch creation is associated with many advantages. Some of these are general to colorectal resections but some such as improved fecundity are unique to the ileoanal pouch. There is a learning curve attached to minimally invasive ileoanal pouch surgery and this chapter aims to discuss technical issues relating to minimally invasive creation of ileoanal pouches and discuss newer approaches.

**Keywords** Laparoscopy · Ileoanal pouch · Transanal surgery · Single incision surgery

## 5.1 Introduction

The efficacy and safety of minimally invasive techniques in both benign and malignant colorectal surgery is now well established and has been adopted widely internationally. The benefits of minimally invasive surgery including reduced blood loss, faster recovery of bowel function, reduced post-operative opioid requirements, reduced wound complications, better cosmesis, earlier discharge, reduced adhesions and reduced rate of incisional hernias can also be achieved with ileoanal pouch surgery [1–5].

The adoption of minimally invasive techniques in pouch surgery has been slower than in other areas of colorectal surgery due to the perceived complexity of the operation, steep learning curve and the lack of evidence in large volume, randomised studies [6]. Despite the lack of evidence, many patients, in particular young patients, the cohort in which this procedure is most prevalent, tend to request a minimally invasive approach probably related to the cosmetic benefits associated with the procedure. Minimally invasive pouch surgery may also result in higher fertility rates in women compared to traditional open pouch surgery [7].

---

N. Hodges · J. Warusavitarne (✉)
St. Mark's Hospital, Harrow, UK
e-mail: Nicola.hodges@nhs.net; j.warusavitarne@nhs.net



J. Warusavitarne, Z. Perry-Woodford (eds.), *The Ileoanal Pouch*,
https://doi.org/10.1007/978-3-319-94385-5_5

## 5.2 Definition

The term minimally invasive pouch surgery is used to describe procedures completed laparoscopically either with the use of multi-port laparoscopy, single incision laparoscopic surgery (SILS), robotic assistance, hand assistance and also includes the more recently described transanal rectal excision techniques.

## 5.3 Patient Selection

The selection of patients with Ulcerative Colitis (UC) or Familial Adenomatous Polyposis (FAP) appropriate for restorative proctocolectomy with ileoanal pouch formation is covered in detail in other chapters of this book. There are no absolute contraindications to a minimally invasive approach provided the surgeon has the appropriate experience and training. There is a suggestion in the literature that patients operated on in high volume pouch centres may experience better immediate and long term outcomes than those who have procedures performed in low volume centres [8]. Patients who have previously had open surgery may have significant adhesions making a minimally invasive approach more challenging and necessitate subsequent conversion to an open procedure but this should not preclude attempting a minimally invasive approach.

## 5.4 Procedure

### *5.4.1 Positioning/Equipment/Port Placement*

As with all laparoscopic surgery, patient positioning, port placement and having appropriate equipment readily available is essential to a successful operation. The patient should be placed in the modified Lloyd Davis position and appropriate manoeuvres to avoid slippage from the bed have to be taken. The arms are placed at the sides and appropriate compression stockings and pneumatic calf compression devices attached. They should be secured with either a suction bean bag device or shoulder/arm supports to allow steep changes of position during the procedure without any risk to nerve injury or the patient slipping on the table. Care needs to be taken to avoid having the supports projecting too high up from the bed as this can interfere with instrument positioning during laparoscopic dissection. An adequate high definition camera system with either a 30° or flexible tipped camera scope is essential with access to multiple video screens/slave monitors. Port positioning is dependent on the approach being taken and will vary depending on surgeon preference. The combined transanal single port approach is becoming a popular approach and is now well described in the literature (Table 5.1 and Figs. 5.1, 5.2 and 5.3).

Standard set up and port placements are shown in the Figs. 5.2 and 5.3. If a combined trans-abdominal/trans-anal approach is being taken we recommend having two theatre teams working simultaneously (see Fig. 5.1).

**Table 5.1** Summary of the current evidence for minimally invasive pouch surgery

| Journal article | Conclusions |
|---|---|
| **Laparoscopic IPAA** | |
| Larson DW, Cima RR, Dozois EJ et al. Safety, feasibility and short-term outcomes of laparoscopic ileal-pouch-anal anastomosis. *Ann. Surg.* 2006; 243: 667–72 | Single institution case-matched<br>100 lap IPAA vs 200 open IPAA<br>90 day follow-up<br>Morbidity equivalent<br>Longer operative time lap. Group<br>Laparoscopic group shorter time to normal diet, reduced post-operative length of stay, shorter time to stoma function and reduced opiate use |
| Ahmed Ali U, Keus F, Heikens JT et al. Open versus laparoscopic (assisted) ileo pouch anal anastomosis for ulcerative colitis and familial adenomatous polyposis. *Cochrane Database Syst. Rev.* 2009: CD006267 | Lap. IPAA feasible and safe procedure<br>No significant difference in mortality or complication rates between the two groups<br>Operative time longer in laparoscopic group |
| El-Gazzaz G.S, Kiran R.P., Remzi F.H. et al. Outcomes for case-matched laparoscopically versus open proctocolectomy. BJS 2009; 96: 522–526 | Retrospective study<br>119 patients lap. Assisted IPAA compared to 238 patients open IPAA<br>5 year follow-up<br>Similar long term outcomes<br>Lap. Group shorter hospital stay and shorter time to onset of stoma function |
| Fajardo et al. Laparoscopic versus open 2-stage ileal pouch: Laparoscopic approach allows for faster restoration of intestinal continuity. J. Am Coll Surg 2010; 211: 377–383 | Retrospective review<br>55 laparoscopic, 69 open IPAA<br>Laparoscopic longer operative time<br>No significant difference in complications<br>Laparoscopic group shorter time to closure of ileostomy |
| Bartels et al. Significantly increased pregnancy rates after laparoscopic restorative proctocolectomy – A cross-sectional study. Ann Surg 2012; 256: 1045–1048 | Retrospective review<br>Higher pregnancy rate in females after laparoscopic IPAA compared with open IPAA |
| Baek et al. Safety, feasibility and short term outcomes in 588 patients undergoing minimally invasive ileal pouch anal anastomosis: a single institution experience. *Techniques Coloproctology* 2016. 20: 369–374 | Retrospective study<br>Laparoscopic or hand assisted<br>30 day follow-up<br>7% operative re-intervention<br>Operating time reduced with increased experience of operating surgeon |

(continued)

**Table 5.1** (continued)

| Journal article | Conclusions |
|---|---|
| **Trans-anal IPAA** | |
| Overstraeten et al. Transanal versus Transabdominal minimally invasive (completion) Proctectomy with Ileal pouch-anal anastomosis in ulcerative colitis – a comparative study. *Ann Surg* 2017. 266: 878–883 | Retrospective study<br>97 TaIPAA, 119 trans-abdominal IPAA<br>No significant difference operative time<br>Shorter post-operative duration of hospital stay TaIPAA (9.08 days) vs trans-abdominal IPAA (7.34 days)<br>Lower conversion rate TaIPAA versus trans-abdominal IPAA (23.5% vs 5.2%)<br>No significant difference in leak rate/complication rate. |
| **SILS & Trans-anal IPAA** | |
| Leo et al. Initial experience of restorative proctocolectomy for ulcerative colitis by transanal total mesorectal excision and single-incision abdominal laparoscopic surgery. *Colorectal Disease.* 2016. 18: 1162–1166 | 16 patients<br>18.7% conversion rate<br>30 day complication rate 37.5%<br>One anastomotic leak |

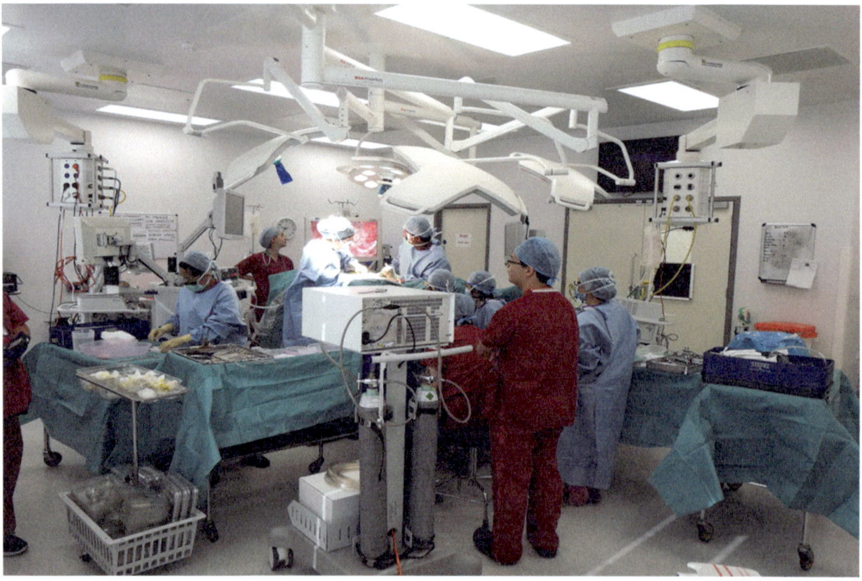

**Fig. 5.1** Operating room set up for the combined single incision/transanal ileoanal pouch operation

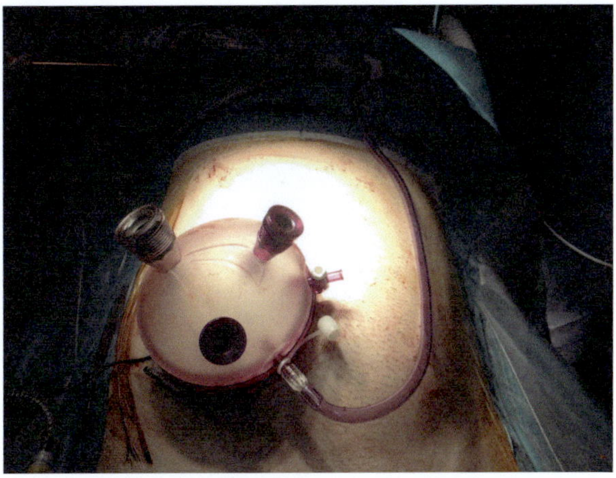

**Fig. 5.2** The port placement in single incision ileoanal pouch surgery with the port placed at the site of the ileotomy

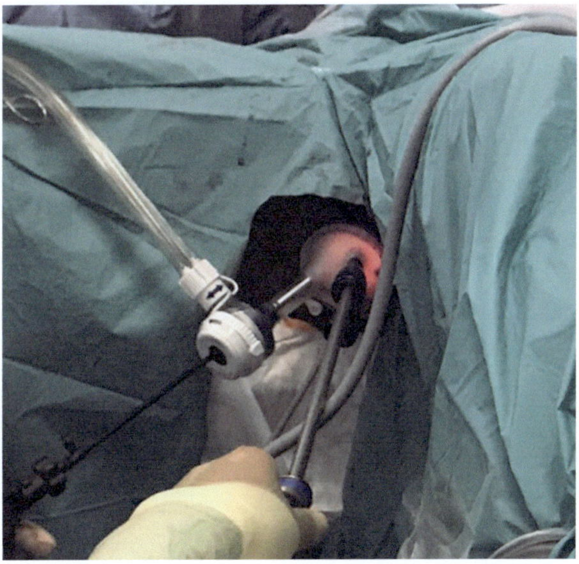

**Fig. 5.3** Transanal port set up for transanal rectal resection

## *5.4.2 Colectomy for Acute UC or Medically Refractory UC*

The rationale for not performing a single stage pouch procedure especially in ulcerative colitis are described in subsequent chapters but it is the authors' preference to perform a subtotal colectomy as the initial operation laparoscopically both in the emergency and semi-elective setting There is much debate on the appropriate

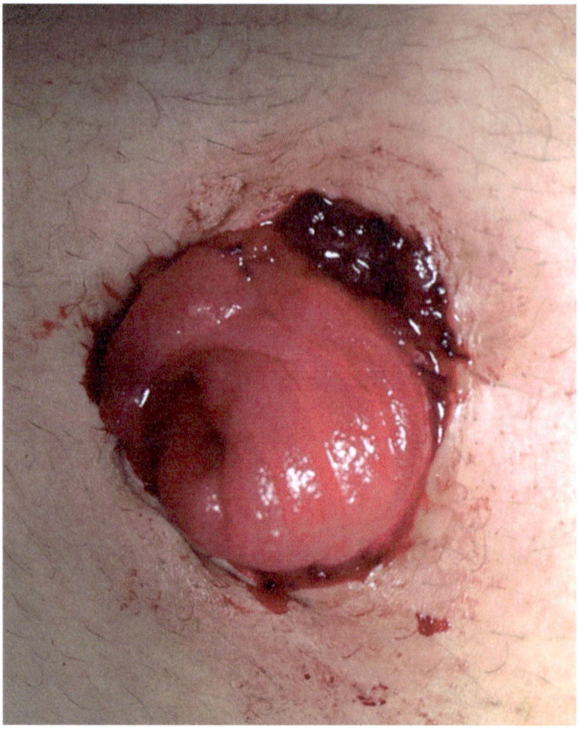

**Fig. 5.4** The mucus fistula is seen placed above and to the left of the ilestomy

management of the rectal stump after colectomy. The rectal stump can be placed intraperitoneally, subcutaneously or as a mucus fistula. The risk of stump blow out is reported to be low but the consequences can be significant given that these patients are immunocompromised [9, 10]. Many of these data originate from audits carried out before the era of biologic drugs in management of acute flares in ulcerative colitis and no risk factors for stump blow out have been described. On this basis it is the authors' preference to exteriorise the rectal stump as a mucus fistula adjacent to the stoma through the same trephine. (see Fig. 5.4). In the event that the rectal stump is left intraperitoneally it is suggested that the inferior mesenteric pedicle is not divided to ensure that the rectal stump does not adhere in the pelvis making subsequent dissection more difficult. There is no evidence to suggest that a short rectal stump has any benefit over a longer stump and we do not recommend this practice as it makes subsequent rectal dissection more challenging.

### 5.4.3 *Proctectomy and Ileoanal Pouch Formation*

Both proctectomy in the TME plane and close rectal dissection have been described in the literature and are used widely, both in the setting of prophylactic surgery for FAP and Ulcerative Colitis. The rationale for close rectal dissection being the potential reduction in autonomic nerve injury. Some also argue that close rectal dissection has other advantages such as better pouch function and reduced pelvic sepsis. (see Chap. 6 by Bemelman). We routinely perform rectal dissection in the TME plane in patients in whom we are performing an ileoanal pouch as we find this plane results in less bleeding. In this plane the hypogastric nerves can be visualised and carefully preserved. Care must be taken not to injure the nerves in both approaches particularly laterally and anteriorly. It can be difficult to advance the pouch to the pelvic floor in the setting of a bulky residual mesorectum following a close rectal dissection and we have concerns about pouch distension and subsequent pouch function in this setting. Given the lack of evidence for either approach at this stage it is reasonable to suggest an individual surgeons preference on the appropriate dissection of the rectum.

It is essential that the rectum is transected low, aiming for a pouch-anal anastomosis approximately 1 cm above the dentate line. This has traditionally been viewed as the greatest limitation with a trans-abdominal minimally invasive approach. In order to ensure that the rectum is transected at the appropriate level a digital rectal examination should be performed prior to firing the stapler. The Trans-anal proctectomy has the potential advantage of being able to easily identify the height of rectal transection, avoiding multiple firings of the linear stapler to transect the rectum and avoiding crossed staple lines with a double purse-string anastomosis. The single stapled anastomosis has the theoretical advantage of a lower leak rate based on the premise that multiple stapler firings are avoided.

### 5.4.4 Specimen Extraction

A variety of extraction site incisions are described in the literature including a Pfannensteil, periumbilical midline incision or using the SILS port site (usually located at site of previous end ileostomy/future loop ileostomy). Prior to specimen extraction and subsequent ileal pouch formation it is essential that the root of the small bowel mesentery has been mobilised to the third part of the duodenum. Pouch lengthening procedures (as detailed in a the Chap. 4 by Phillips) should also be performed as required to avoid tension on the pouch-anal anastomosis.

### 5.4.5 Pouch Formation

The authors' prefer to perform a 15 cm ileal J pouch with the distal 30 cm of terminal ileum. This is fashioned with 2–3 firings of a linear stapler. The distal end is oversewn and potential points of weakness of staplers which are at the points of initiation of the stapler firings (traditionally called the 'Phillips' points at St. Mark's Hospital after Professor Robin Phillips who described them) are oversewn. A 2-0 prolene purse string suture is placed around the anvil of a 29/31 mm circular stapler. Prior to forming the pouch, it is important to ensure that there is adequate length to reach the anus (this is described in the Chap. 4).

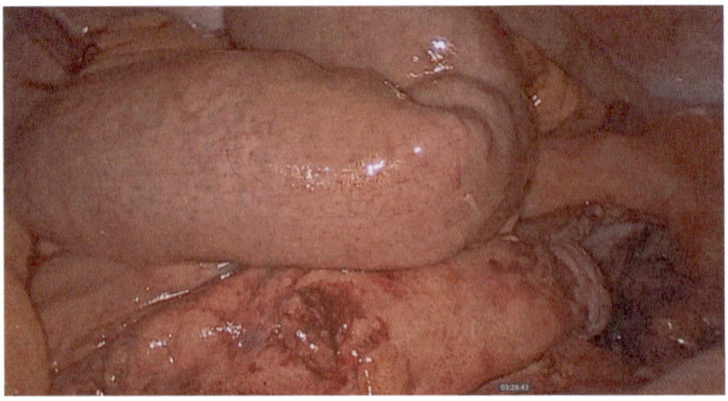

**Fig. 5.5** Small bowel mesentery placed in a straight line on the patients right hand side with all small bowel above and to the left of this

### *5.4.6 Anastomosis*

Prior to performing the circular stapled anastomosis care needs to be taken to ensure there is no twisting of the pouch during advancement to the pelvic floor and that the mesentery of the small bowel can be followed and is straight from D3 to the anastomosis without loops of small bowel herniating underneath. The most effective method for ensuring there is no twist in the pouch is to tilt the patient in the right side up position and allow all the small bowel to migrate to the left of the abdominal cavity. The small bowel is then unravelled if needed and the mesenteric edge is visualised to ensure that no small bowel is to the right side of the mesentery or under the mesentery. Once this has been achieved the bowel can be exteriorised to form the pouch and subsequently returned to the peritoneal cavity with the patient in the same position. Again, when the pouch is lowered to the pelvis, the mesenteric edge should always be visualised to ensure the pouch is not twisted during the anastomosis (see Fig. 5.5).

### *5.4.7 Ileostomy Formation*

Whether or not the pouch-anal anastomosis is defunctioned with a temporary loop ileostomy is up to the operating surgeon. Traditionally a defunctioning ileostomy would be performed routinely apart from in such cases in which there isn't adequate length to bring out a stoma through the abdominal wall without placing too much tension on the pouch anal anastomosis. Routinely this would be placed in the right iliac fossa at site of previous end ileostomy but in some cases the left side may need to be used. The balance of risks between the potential morbidity of an ileostomy versus those of an uncovered pouch need to be considered.

## 5.5 Post Operative Management

We would advocate the use of an enhanced recovery after surgery (ERAS) protocol. Care needs to be taken to monitor the patient closely in the early post-operative period and consider CT scanning early to detect possible leak/peri-pouch collection in order to achieve drainage as soon as possible (see Chap. 6 by Bemelman).

## 5.6 Investigations Prior to Closure of Ileostomy

All patients should have a water soluble contrast enema to assess the integrity of the pouch and pouch-anal anastomosis prior to closure of ileostomy in addition to a thorough examination under anaesthesia at the time of closure of ileostomy. Any pouch-anal anastomotic stricture should be dilated in order to enable passage of the surgeons index finger prior to closing the ileostomy.

## 5.7 Considerations

Although we advocate the use of minimally invasive techniques in ileoanal pouch surgery and the adoption of such techniques is becoming more widespread it must be emphasised again, the paucity of quality randomised trials in the literature relating to these techniques. Although laparoscopic techniques appear to be safe when compared to the open approach, a clear superiority, in terms of complications and long term function pouch and sexual function has not been proven. Operative times are significantly longer in laparoscopic compared to open groups [11–17]. Larger, prospective, randomised studies are still required. In particular long term functional outcomes in those patients who have undergone a trans-anal approach have not been assessed. It also needs to be remembered that the minimally invasive approach is not suitable for all patients/surgeons. Particular consideration needs to be given to FAP patients with desmoidogenic mutations as data from the Cleveland clinic suggests a higher rate of desmoid formation following laparoscopic versus open proctocolectomy and IPAA (This has been discussed in detail in the Chap. 10 by Clark) [18].

## References

1. Lacy AM, Garcia-Valdecasas JC, Delgado S, et al. Laparoscopy-assisted colectomy versus open colectomy for treatment of non-metastatic colon cancer: a randomised trial. Lancet. 2002;359:2224–9.

2. Guillou PJ, Quirke P, Thorpe H, et al. Short-term endpoints of conventional versus laparoscopic-assisted surgery in patients with colorectal cancer (MRC CLASICC trial): multicentre randomised controlled trial. Lancet. 2005;365:1718–26.
3. Clinical Outcomes of Surgical Therapy Study Group. A comparison of laparoscopically assisted and open colectomy for colon cancer. N Engl J Med. 2004;350:2050–9.
4. Veldkamp R, Kuhry E, Hop WC, et al. Laparoscopic surgery versus open surgery for colon cancer: short term outcomes of a randomised trial. Lancet Oncol. 2005;6:477–84.
5. Vlug MS, Wind J, Hollmann MW, et al. Laparoscopy in combination with fast track multimodal management is the best perioperative strategy in patients undergoing colonic surgery: a randomised clinical trial (LAFA-study). Ann Surg. 2011;254:868–75.
6. Hemandas A, Jenkins J. Laparoscopic pouch surgery in ulcerative colitis. Ann Gastroenterol. 2012;25:309–16.
7. Bartels SA, et al. Significantly increased pregnancy rates after laparoscopic restorative proctocolectomy – a cross-sectional study. Ann Surg. 2012;256:1045–8.
8. Burns EM, Bottle A, Aylin P, et al. Volume analysis of outcome following restorative proctocolectomy. Br J Surg. 2011;98:408–17.
9. Gu J, Stocchi L, Remzi F, Kiran RP. Intraperitoneal or subcutaneous: does location of the (colo)rectal stump influence outcomes after laparoscopic total abdominal colectomy for ulcerative colitis? Dis Colon Rectum. 2013;56:615–21.
10. Brady RR, Collie MH, Ho GT, et al. Outcomes of the rectal remnant following colectomy for ulcerative colitis. Colorectal Dis. 2008;10:144–50.
11. Larson DW, Cima RR, Dozois EJ, et al. Safety, feasibility and short-term outcomes of laparoscopic ileal-pouch-anal anastomosis. Ann Surg. 2006;243:667–72.
12. Ahmed Ali U, Keus F, Heikens JT, et al. Open versus laparoscopic (assisted) ileo pouch anal anastomosis for ulcerative colitis and familial adenomatous polyposis. Cochrane Database Syst Rev. 2009:CD006267.
13. El-Gazzaz GS, Kiran RP, Remzi FH, et al. Outcomes for case-matched laparoscopically versus open proctocolectomy. BJS. 2009;96:522–6.
14. Fajardo AD, et al. Laparoscopic versus open 2-stage ileal pouch: laparoscopic approach allows for faster restoration of intestinal continuity. J Am Coll Surg. 2010;211:377–83.
15. Baek SJ, et al. Safety, feasibility and short term outcomes in 588 patients undergoing minimally invasive ileal pouch anal anastomosis: a single institution experience. Tech Coloproctol. 2016;20:369–74.
16. de Buck van Overstraeten A, et al. Transanal versus transabdominal minimally invasive (completion) proctectomy with ileal pouch-anal anastomosis in ulcerative colitis – a comparative study. Ann Surg. 2017;266:878–83.
17. Leo CA, et al. Initial experience of restorative proctocolectomy for ulcerative colitis by transanal total mesorectal excision and single-incision abdominal laparoscopic surgery. Colorectal Dis. 2016;18:1162–6.
18. Vogel JCJ, LaGuardia L. Minimally invasive pouch surgery predisposes to desmoid tumour formation in patients with familial adenomatous polyposis. *The American Society of Colon and Rectal Surgeons Annual Meeting Abstracts, April 30-May 5, 2005, Philadelphia Pennysylvania.* Philadelphia. Dis Colon Rectum. 2005;662

# Chapter 6
# The Complicated Pouch

**Willem A. Bemelman, Karin A. T. G. M. Wasmann, Christianne J. Buskens, and Pieter J. Tanis**

**Abstract** Restorative proctocolectomy and reconstruction with an ileoanal pouch offers select patients some advantages over permanent ileostomy. Complications can occur intraoperatively or in the early or late phases post-operatively, which may have devastating effects on patient outcomes and quality of life. Early detection of complications and multidisciplinary management in centres with sufficient expertise is vital for pouch salvage.

**Keywords** Early salvage · Late salvage · Inflammatory dysfunction · Mechanical dysfunction · Management techniques · Expertise · Quality of life

## 6.1 Introduction

Restorative proctocolectomy and reconstruction with an ileoanal pouch is the procedure of choice in patients with ulcerative colitis and may be required in some patients with polyposis coli (see Chap. 3). The most well-known pouch configurations are the J-, the S- and the W-pouch (Fig. 6.1a–c). Alternative designs have been J-like pouches with multiple septa, (the B-pouch), hypothesizing that the septa would prevent stasis in the pouch resulting in less pouchitis.

Over time, cumulative evidence demonstrated that the J-pouch is the superior pouch, because off its relatively ease of construction, and its superiority in emptying compared to the S-, and W-pouches [1, 2]. Thus far, there is no consensus on the ideal length of a J-pouch, but most surgeons would make a pouch with a length of 10–20 cm.

The reservoirs could be stapled to the anus using the double stapling technique leaving a small rim of rectal mucosa called "the cuff", or applying a handsewn technique mostly in combination with a mucosectomy. Mucosectomy is particularly advocated in patients with polyposis coli to remove all polyp bearing mucosa.

W. A. Bemelman (✉) · K. A. T. G. M. Wasmann · C. J. Buskens · P. J. Tanis
Department of Surgery, Amsterdam, The Netherlands
e-mail: w.a.bemelman@amc.nl; k.a.wasmann@amc.nl; c.j.buskens@amc.nl; p.j.tanis@amc.nl



J. Warusavitarne, Z. Perry-Woodford (eds.), *The Ileoanal Pouch*,
https://doi.org/10.1007/978-3-319-94385-5_6

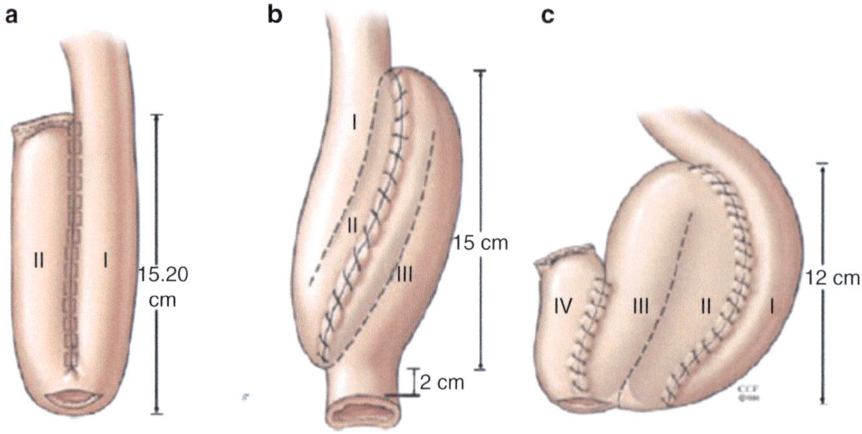


**Fig. 6.1** (**a**) J-pouch (**b**) S-pouch (**c**) W-pouch. (Reprinted with permission from the Cleveland clinic [3])

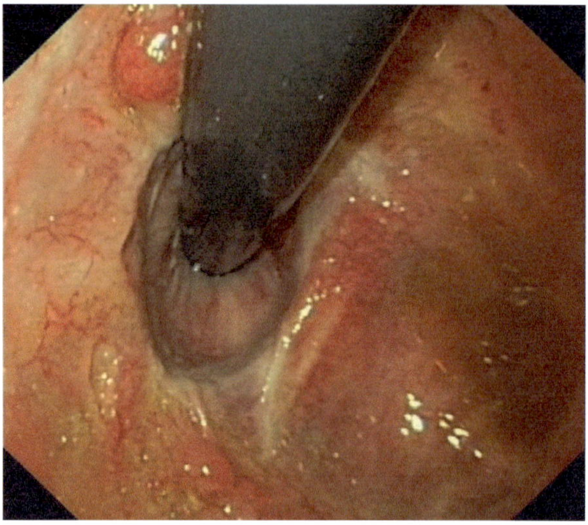

**Fig. 6.2** Double stapled anastomosis with rectal cuff in retroversion

Studies comparing stapling versus handsewn in combination with mucosectomy, showed an increased incidence of nocturnal soiling and anastomotic stenosis in patients with handsewn anastomosis [2, 4–6]. The current standard for most surgeons is to perform a stapled ileoanal J-pouch reservoir with a remaining rectal cuff of less than 2 cm (Fig. 6.2). If the cuff is longer than 2 cm, the remaining rectum is called "retained rectum", which must be considered a technical error.

There are different strategies used in performing restorative proctocolectomy:

1. One stage: restorative proctocolectomy and pouch is performed in one stage, without the creation of a diverting ileostomy.

2. Two stage: a restorative proctocolectomy and pouch is done with defunctioning ileostomy in the first stage. In a second stage the stoma is closed.
3. Three stage: subtotal colectomy with end-ileostomy in the first stage, followed by completion proctocolectomy and pouch with defunctioning ileostomy in the second stage. In a third staged the stoma is reversed.
4. Modified two stage: subtotal colectomy with end-ileostomy first, followed by completion proctocolectomy and pouch without an ileostomy in the second stage.

The one and two stage procedures are preserved for polyposis coli patients who are generally fit and healthy patients. The three and modified two stage procedures are performed in ulcerative colitis patients, as they can be immunocompromised (medication related)), are malnourished and/or anaemic. Combined data of three referral institutes showed that defunctioning the pouch in these patients (two stage) is ineffective in preventing anastomotic leakage and is associated with long-term complications, while the modified two stage enables the patients to wean off the drugs and recover resulting in lower leak rates. For this reason, a modified 2-stage or three stage procedure is preferred for UC [7–9].

In most situations ideally, the colectomy should be carried out laparoscopically [10]. In the second stage, the proctocolectomy and pouch construction can be performed either via a Pfannenstiel incision or via single port and Transanal minimally invasive surgery (TAMIS). The first results of the latter showed improved perioperative outcomes [9]. It is hypothesized TAMIS results in better outcomes due to improved visualization and accessibility of the pelvis and rectum which eases the proctectomy and facilitates a close rectal dissection. Performing the dissection close to the bowel wall reduces the risk of autonomic nerve lesions, preventing iatrogenic urinary and sexual dysfunction. Other proposed advantages are the preservation of the posterior mesorectal fat which might be associated with a lower rate of local septic complications, presacral hematoma or abscess [11]. Furthermore, it is suggested that by preserving the mesorectum and its nerves, a greater awareness of pouch filling is achieved compared to removing the mesorectum, probably due to different proprioception [12]. Using the TAMIS technique the difficult double stapling is no longer necessary, and is replaced by a single stapled anastomosis [13].

Pouch surgery is specialized surgery and institutional volume is important in reducing complications. High institutional volume is associated with decreased complications, and enables units to handle early and late complications better. For this reason, the Surgical Committee of the European Crohn's and Colitis Organisation (S-ECCO) guidelines on Ulcerative Colitis state that pouch surgery should be only done in units where more than 10 procedures per year are performed [14]. This figure must be considered as a starting point to encourage surgeons and national bodies to centralize pouch surgery instead of performing a small number annually.

## 6.2 Complications

Complications can be separated into early and late complications.

## 6.2.1 *Early Salvage*

### 6.2.1.1 Endosponge Treatment

The Achilles heel of pouch surgery is the ileoanal anastomosis. Leak rates of the different series vary from 2.3% to 26.7%, depending on the staging and follow-up [15]. Combined series of three tertiary referral hospitals showed a leak rate of 18% [7].

The traditional management of the early leak is to defunction the leak, (if not carried out at the index operation) and observe the outcome. In case of big abscesses transanal irrigation with a catheter can be performed (Fig. 6.3). This results in a long period before the abscess heals, and within that time period some of the abscesses can progress to a persistent presacral sinus. Prior or persistent leaks of the ileoanal pouch are the most important cause of long term pouch failure and should therefore be treated aggressively [16–18].

Weidenhagen et al. proposed in 2008 a vacuum assisted drainage of the cavity using an endosponge placed endoscopically via the defect in the anastomosis into

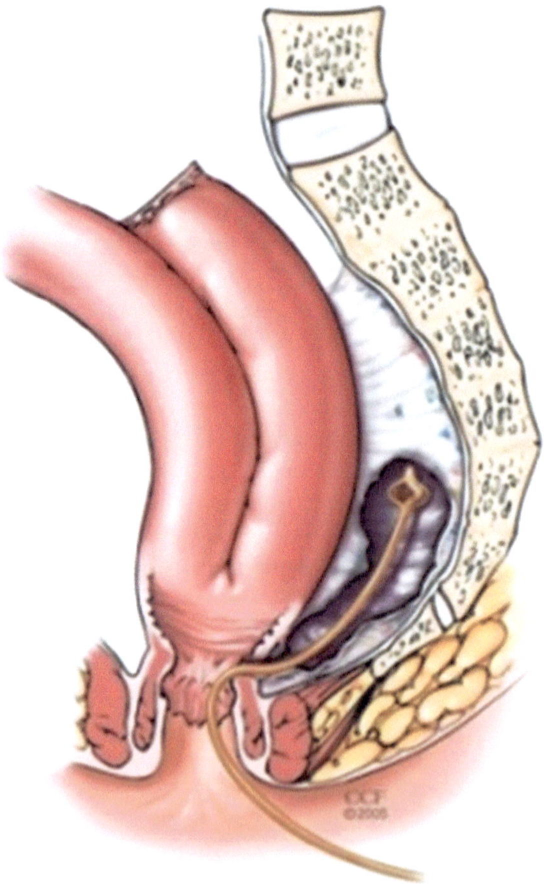


**Fig. 6.3** Conventional management of anastomotic leak [21]

the cavity [19]. This endosponge connected to a 150 mm Hg vacuum bottle ensured an active drainage of the abscess cavity (Figs. 4.1 and 4.2). Endosponge changes need to be carried iut every 3–4 days under light sedation in the endoscopy room to prevent tissue ingrowth in the endosponge. By gradually tapering the size of the endosponge, the collapsed cavity was replaced by the neorectum. Weidenhagen described this technique for colorectal and coloanal anastomosis. Gardenbroek et al. from the Amsterdam group described an adaptation of this technique, applying the endosponge for pouch leaks [20]. The endosponge was only used for cleansing of the cavity, and after two or three placements the patient was brought back to surgery to close the defect at the anastomosis.

#### 6.2.1.2 Anastomotic Closure

When the abscess cavity is considered clean and the edges of the anastomosis were mobile, the anastomotic defect can be closed surgically. Under general anesthesia the patient is placed in the Lloyd Davis position. Following, a pudendal nerve block is given bilaterally. Extraction of the endosponge is done after flushing the tubing with saline in order to facilitate the sponge extraction and prevent bleeding from the cavity. In general, the pouch anal anastomosis low enough for the anastomosis to be exposed using retractors, facilitated by the Lonestar retractor. Next, the cavity is irrigated with saline. A small drain is positioned in the cavity, which is brought outside through the sphincter muscle, hence outside the anastomotic defect, and is connected to a vacuum bottle. The anastomotic dehiscence is transanally sutured with interrupted 2-0 Vicryl using a small curved needle. The vacuum drain is removed on the third postoperative day and patients are treated with antibiotics for 10 days. Two weeks after closure endoscopy is performed to evaluate whether the closure has been successful. If the anastomosis is intact, a CT scan with intraluminal contrast is ordered to confirm this finding. In case of failure, the endosponge placement and surgical closure can be attempted a second time, or the original Weidenhagen technique can be applied tapering the endosponge over a number of weeks to close the cavity. So far, this endosponge treatment and surgical closure resulted in a 100% closure of 15 leaking ileoanal pouches in a much shorter time than the traditional wait and see and/or irrigation approach [20]. Early detection and initiation of the endosponge technique is crucial for successful closure, and probably avoids the negative sequelae of anastomotic leakage on pouch function. Future data are awaited with respect to long term outcome.

The perioperative management after pouch construction can be as follows:

1. Ileoanal pouch with defunctioning stoma:

   Standard CRP measurement at day 4, if >140 a CT scan with rectal contrast is indicated. In case of leakage, endosponge placement in the endoscopy department should be performed, the additional endosponge treatment should be executed as described above. Pinpoint defects must first be dilated to 12 mm to facilitate the over tube required to insert the endosponge.

If at day 4 the CRP < 140 and the patient is in clinical good condition, pouchoscopy is performed after 2 weeks to inspect the defunctioned anastomosis for integrity. Check for pus evacuation, bubbles and granuloma on the anastomotic site. In case of leak start with endosponge treatment.

2. Ileoanal pouch without defunctioning stoma:

   Most units would decompress the pouch with a pouch drain for several days and put the patient on a fluid diet. The day before and the day after the pouch drain has been removed a CRP is taken. If CRP is >140, a CT scan with rectal contrast must be performed. In case of a leak, the patient is brought back to surgery to create a defunctioning ileostomy and to insert the first endosponge. After 1–2 endosponge exchanges the defect in the anastomosis is surgically closed (Fig. 6.4).

### 6.2.2 *Late Salvage of the Dysfunctioning Pouch*

Causes for late pouch dysfunction can be subdivided into mechanical and inflammatory/septic. The symptoms are high stool frequency initiated by either, mechanical emptying problems resulting in paradoxal diarrhea or inflammatory septic problems resulting in a lower pouch compliance. Mechanical causes include

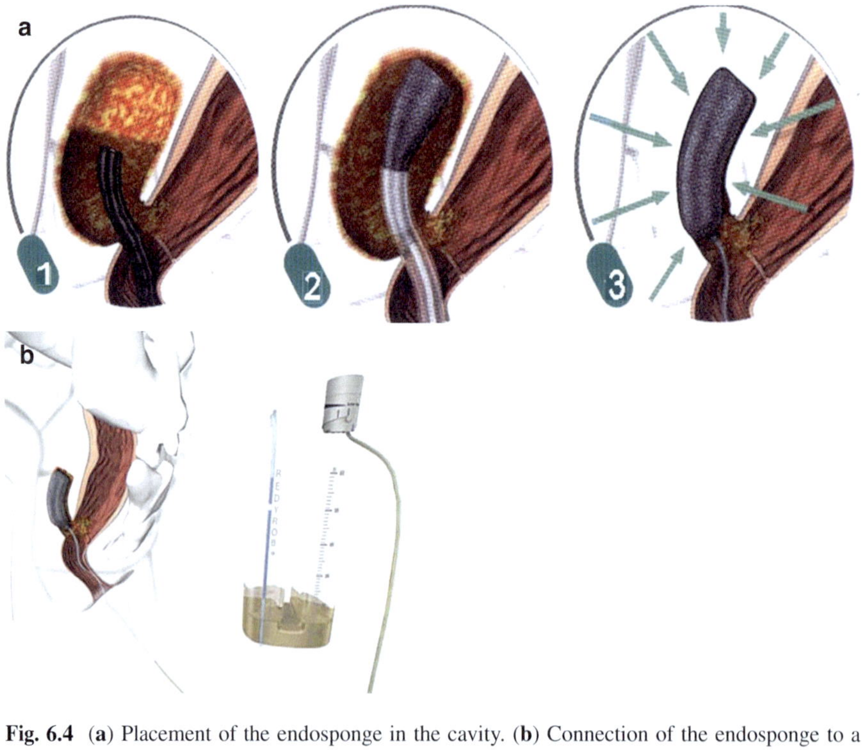


**Fig. 6.4** (**a**) Placement of the endosponge in the cavity. (**b**) Connection of the endosponge to a low-vacuum suction bottle. (Reprinted with permission from B-Braun)

strictures of the anastomosis, afferent and efferent loop syndrome, torsion of the pouch, intussusception and prolapse of the pouch, redundant blind loop and mega-pouch. Inflammatory/septic causes include late leaks manifested as presacral abscesses and anastomotic vaginal fistula, cuffitis, retained rectum, and Crohn's disease.

Diagnostics always include pouchoscopy, preferably carried out by the gastroenterologist and surgeon together since interpretation of the pouchoscopy can be difficult. In addition, cross-sectional imaging by CT scan with intraluminal contrast or pelvic MRI must be done to assess pouch size, to evaluate the afferent and efferent loop, and determine the presence of a presacral sinus. When there is a suspicion of emptying problems, defecography or dynamic pelvic MRI are helpful to assess what is going on during defecation.

## 6.3 Mechanical Causes of Dysfunction

(a) Anastomotic stricture:

Anastomotic stricture of the pouch anal anastomosis is mostly seen in patients with handsewn anastomosis or in patients after a healed anastomotic leakage [2]. These persistent strictures are unlike those seen in defunctioned double stapling line strictures that can easily be dilated with the finger. Anastomotic strictures can be treated with dilatation using Hegar dilators. Typically, the first dilatation is performed under general anesthesia aiming at a diameter of at least 1 cm. Thereafter, the patient can maintain the effect by self-dilatation. If this is not successful, the stricture needs to be excised and a pouch sleeve advancement must be done with hand sewn anastomosis. In case the stricture has been present for a long time, the pouch can be dilated in such a way that emptying problems might persist, despite having a patent anastomosis. Subsequently, remodeling the pouch into a smaller size is sometimes necessary.

(b) Afferent loop syndrome:

The afferent loop syndrome is a situation where the afferent loop to the pouch is kinking behind the pouch precluding filling of the pouch. The patient has obstructive symptoms. The diagnosis is made by MRI or CT-scan. The solution is to lyse the small bowel loop from the pelvis, fill the space behind the pouch with omentum if present, and fix the bowel loop with sutures to prevent falling behind the pouch. This can be performed laparoscopically (Fig. 6.5a–d).

(c) Efferent loop syndrome:

The efferent loop is exclusively associated with S-pouches with a efferent loop that is too long, causing kinking of the efferent loop during defecation. Most of the S-pouches were created in the 90s and thus this is now rarely seen. When constructing the S-pouch, the efferent loop must be no longer than 2 cm. A efferent loop that is too long with a kink, might cause evacuation problems with gradual dilatation of the pouch and increasingly paradoxical diarrhea. If

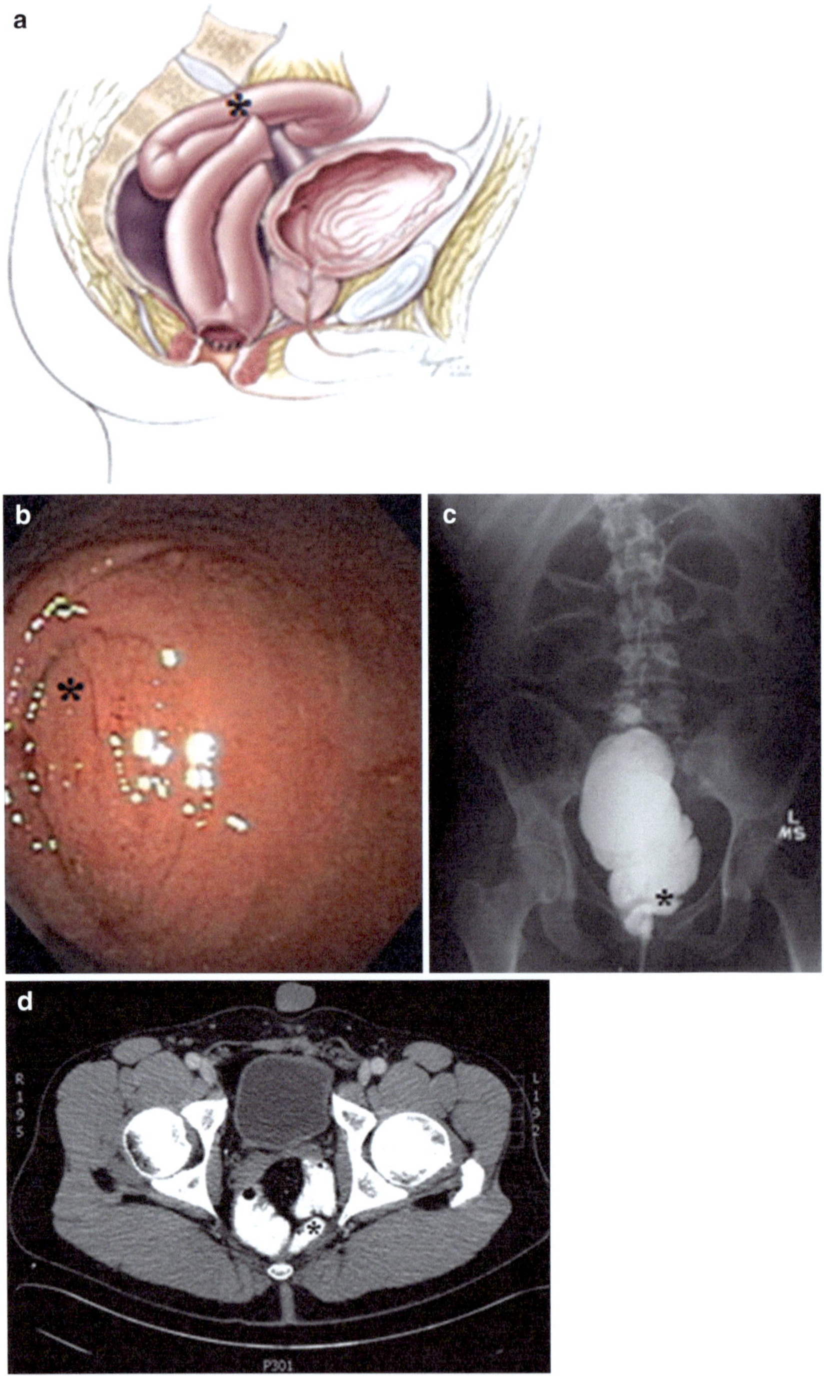


**Fig. 6.5** (**a**) Schematic representation of the afferent loop herniated behind the pouch (*). (**b**, **c**) show the endoscopic and the radiologic picture of the kinked afferent loop (*). (**d**) depicts a CT scan which shows the afferent loop behind the pouch [21]. (Reprinted with permission from Liska et al. [21])

a patient presents with a history of increasing emptying problems when having a S-pouch, the most common cause is a kinking efferent loop with gradual expansion of the pouch. The diagnosis is made by defecography, endoscopy and pelvic MRI. The initial approach to the problem is, transanal excision of the redundant efferent loop and creating a new handsewn anastomosis between the body of the pouch and the anus. If this does not improve emptying, despite a patent anastomosis directly to the body of the pouch, it might be necessary to revise the pouch by making the pouch smaller (Fig. 6.6).

(d) Torsion of the pouch or afferent loop

Torsion of the pouch or afferent loop is a diagnosis mostly made on the basis of the patient's history and endoscopic findings. The patient complains of intermittent abdominal cramps and is unable the defecate. Quite often they report that manipulation of the abdomen or change of position will result in a defecation. Endoscopic findings in acute obstruction are a functional stenosis of the afferent loop to the pouch which can be passed easily with the endoscope. Leaving a temporary canula in the afferent loop might solve the acute obstruction. Fixation of the afferent pouch mesentery and bowel loop to the posterior abdominal wall with sutures might prevent recurrent torsion. Another option is to fix the afferent loop to the anterior abdominal wall. In our experience, the torsion of the pouch typically occurs in patients who have no adhesions and a lax mesentery. Despite suturing the afferent loop and its mesentery, the torsion tends to recur, because the fixation sutures gradually wear out on the long term. The ultimate fixation of the afferent loop is to defunction the pouch with an ileostomy.

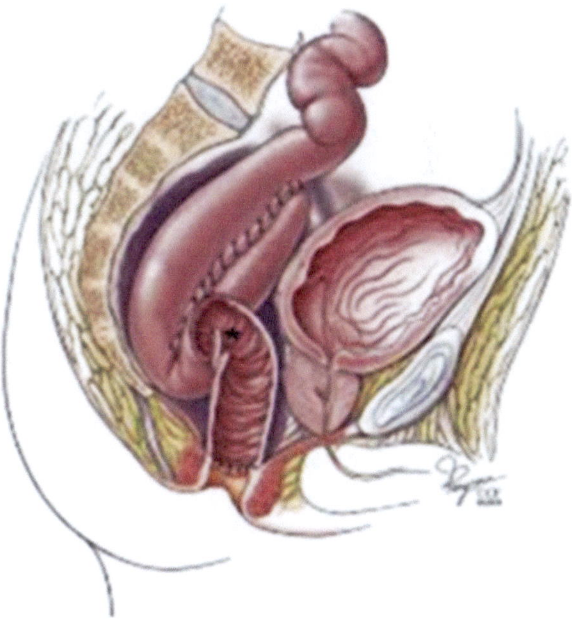

**Fig. 6.6** Schematic representation of a S-pouch with its efferent loop (*) [21]

(e) Redundant blind loop

The redundant blind loop is typically a problem of the J-pouch. If the blind loop of the J-pouch is not kept short and incorporated into the pouch body, the blind loop can gently expand, causing stasis, bacterial overgrowth, and pouchitis. The blind loop can be incorporated in the pouch using a transanally advanced linear endostapler. A more invasive alternative is to dissect and resect the redundant blind loop (Fig. 6.7).

(f) Pouch prolapse

Pouch prolapse is a rare (Fig. 6.8). In the literature there are a few cases described. The largest series is described by Ehsan et al., comprising 83 pouch prolapses [2]. Symptoms are in line with symptoms of rectal prolapse, e.g. recurrent prolapse with soiling. At reoperation these patients show a remarkable lack of adhesions and often a completely peritonealised pelvis, where the pouch is freely mobile due to a lax and unattached mesentery. Fixation of the pouch (pouchopexy) to the sacrum and pouch mesentery to the posterior abdominal wall with non-resorbable interrupted sutures can be performed laparoscopically due to the absence of adhesions. Alternatively, a biological mesh can be used to fix the pouch. Partial mucosal prolapse may be treated with stool bulking agents or a local perineal procedure [22].

## 6.4 Inflammatory or Septic Causes of Dysfunction

(a) *Late anastomotic leak manifesting as chronic presacral sinus*

Unexplained dysfunction of the pouch warrants cross sectional imaging to look for a presacral sinus. At endoscopy, quite often a small orifice is noticed

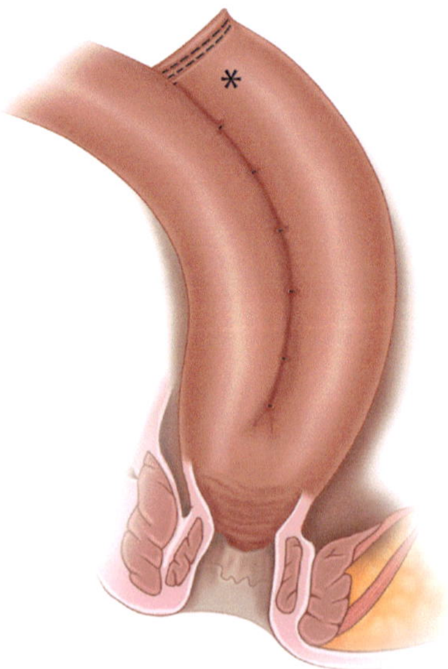


**Fig. 6.7** J-pouch with a blind loop (*). (Permission obtained from K.A. Wasmann)

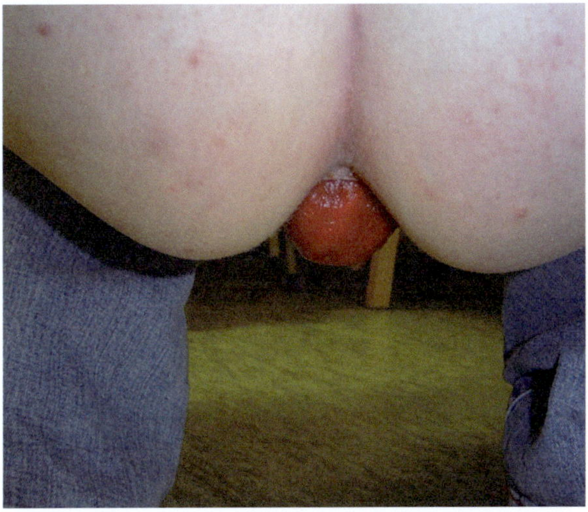

**Fig. 6.8** Full thickness pouch prolapse

where air bubbles or a small amount of pus can be seen. Patients are frequently treated by the gastroenterologist with intermittent courses of antibiotics on the suspicion of having pouchitis. Antibiotics do improve symptoms, but after stopping the antibiotics symptoms will recur, as the underlying cause is not resolved. If the anastomotic insufficiency is small, an attempt can be made to treat the cavity with an endosponge. This often requires dilatation of the defect to facilitate the over tube, necessary to insert the endosponge. Additionally, the pouch needs to be defunctioned. After cleansing of the cavity, the hole in the anastomosis can be closed as described before (Figs. 6.9a–f, and 6.10). This is only possible if the defect is very small, because larger anastomotic insufficiencies are not amenable for suture closure due to retraction and fibrosis of the wall. In this case the patient must be counseled to discuss and decide between a permanent stoma and redo pouch surgery. A permanent defunctioning ileostomy might be sufficient to make the presacral sinus asymptomatic. If the patient is motivated to undergo redo pouch surgery, the pouch can be disconnected from the anus, and mobilized transanally and transabdominally. The tip of the pouch is excised, the septic cavity curetted, and a new ileoanal anastomosis is created. A vulnerable point of the operation is a recurrent abscess in the former cavity perforating through the newly constructed anastomosis resulting in a leak again. Endosponge assisted closure of the defect is an option to solve this problem. If the patient does not want a redo pouch and the presacral sinus causes problems, e.g. intermittent pelvic sepsis or foul discharge of pus, an intersphincteric pouch excision with permanent end-ileostomy can be done in a combined transanal and transabdominal approach. It is important not to leave any mucosa behind and to fill the pelvic cavity preferably with omentum. If there is no omentum, the mesentery of the pouch can be used after close bowel excision of the pouch [23]. This is preferable to muscle flap filling of the pelvis because of the donor site morbidity of for instance rectal abdominal muscle flaps. The feared complication is a persistent presacral abscess draining via the perineum.

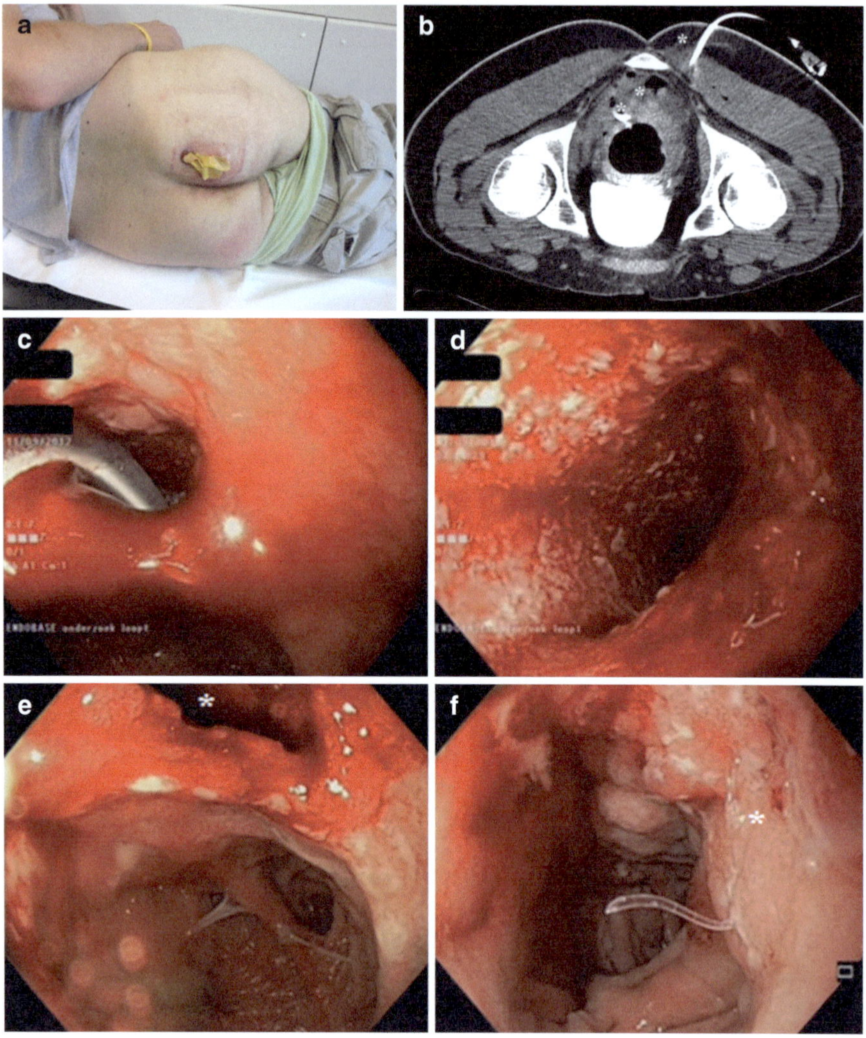

**Fig. 6.9** Patient with chronic presacral abscess due to anastomotic leakage (**a**) percutaneous drainage of presacral abscess behind the pouch, (**b**) Patient lying face down, development of fistula between ileoanal anastomosis (*), presacral cavity (*) and buttock after removal of the drain (*) (**c**) endosponge in cavity after diversion, (**d**) clean granulating cavity, (**e**) small anastomotic defect amenable for suturing (*), (**f**) endoscopic evaluation 2 weeks after closure of the anastomotic insufficiency (*)

(b) Anastomotic vaginal fistula

Anastomotic vaginal fistula can occur shortly after the creation of the pouch or as a long term complication (early versus late onset). When it occurs after pouch creation or closure of the defunctioning stoma, it must be considered as a technical error incorporating part of the vaginal wall into the circular stapler.

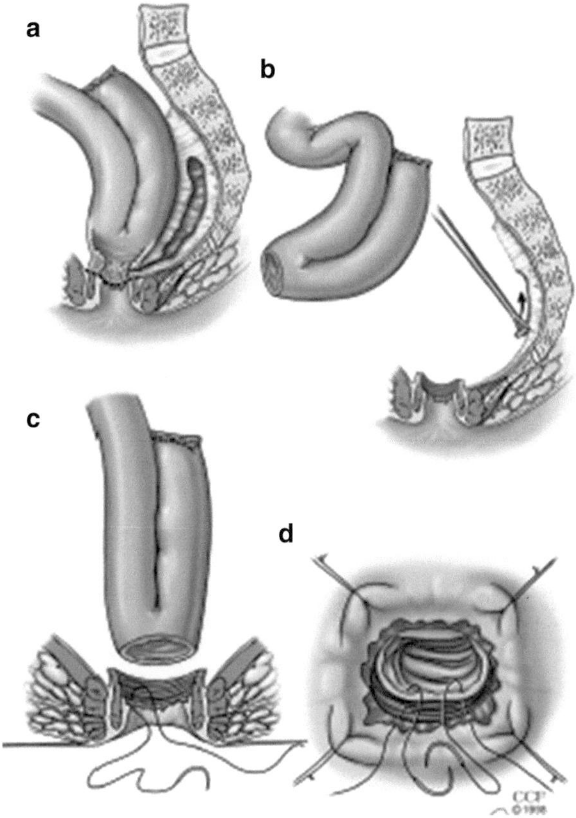


Fig. 6.10 Schematic display with detachment of the pouch, cleansing of the cavity, and restoration of the pouch for pouch recovery after chronic presacral abscess. (Reprinted with permission, Cleveland Clinic Center for Medical Art & Photography)

In relation to late fistulas, Crohn's disease of the cuff or a persistent sinus due to a chronic leak must be ruled out. The rule of thumb is that if symptoms are mild and can be alleviated with stool thickeners, a non-operative approach must be followed. If intermittent rectovaginal septum abscesses are the problem, a seton might provide more optimal drainage. If symptoms are debilitatin, and Crohn's disease is ruled out, surgery aiming at repair can be performed under the protection of a defunctioning ileostomy. A number of options are available, all with moderate success rates varying from partial pouch advancement with anterior sphincter muscle interposition to gracilis muscle interposition. Theodoropoulos et al. described in his systematic review outcomes of ileoanal advancement for pouch vaginal fistula, that approximately half of the patients will benefit from this procedure. Transvaginal repair was associated with a success rate of only 33.3%. Subsequent diagnosis of Crohn's disease and pouch vaginal fistula is prognostic for pouch failure [24, 25].

(c) Cuffitis

Cuffitis refractory to antibiotics and anti-inflammatory suppositories can be excised transanally [26]. Applying the TAMIS technique, the pouch can be mobilized from below [26]. The cuff and the ileoanal anastomosis can be pulled out and resected through the anus. Next, a new hand sewn anastomosis is made. If sufficient, mobilization is achieved to perform the sleeve advancement and anastomosis, this can be done without a transabdominal mobilization and defunctioning ileostomy.

(d) Retained rectum

A retained rectum can become symptomatic if proctitis recurs. After medical therapy fails to control the symptoms, the retained rectum must be excised and the pouch re-anastomosed at an appropriate distance from the anus. A combined transanal and transabdominal approach is required to excise the rectum, mobilize the pouch and lengthen the mesentery to bring down at the pouch. A stapled anastomosis can be performed under these circumstances. A bottom up approach with close rectal dissection, is a very safe and effective way to dissect the pouch rectal anastomosis without damaging the distal pouch, with simultaneous transabdominal top down dissection and rendezvous [27].

(e) Crohn's disease.

In the event of Crohn's disease in the pouch it is generally not advised that any intervention of the pouch other than drainage procedures, defunctioning of the pouch or pouch excision is carried out. Redo surgery aiming at preserving a functional pouch are not associated with successful outcomes [28]. As a first step in debilitating Crohn's disease of the pouch, (e.g. intermittent sepsis with perianal fistula from the pouch) can be defunctioned. Persisting issues not improved by defunctioning are indications for pouch excision.

### 6.4.1 Surgical Approaches

(a) *Transanal excision of cuff, retained rectum or efferent loop and sleeve advancement of the pouch with or without transabdominal mobilization of the pouch.*

All of the following procedures commence by positioning the patient in the Lloyd Davis position, a pudendal nerve block to relax the external sphincter muscle, and application of a Lonestar retractor.

**Cuff/ efferent loop excision** Depending on the level of the anastomosis, either by using separate retractors or the TAMIS platform, the rectal mucosa is incised just below the ileoanal anastomosis (Fig. 6.11 a–c) [26]. If the prior anastomosis was already down to the dentate line (e.g. S-pouch), care should be taken not to damage the internal sphincter. Transection through the muscular wall should be carried out cranial or at the level of the ileoanal anastomosis in order to preserve the internal sphincter muscle. Careful dissection of the distal pouch or the efferent loop is then performed. If mobilization of the distal pouch or efferent loop is very successful, the mobilized part can be exteriorized via the anus, the cuff or efferent loop can be excised and a handsewn anastomosis can be made. If bottom up mobilization is insufficient, either open or laparoscopic mobilization of the proximal part of the pouch and its mesentery must be done. In the latter case, it is advisable to defunction the handsewn anastomosis.

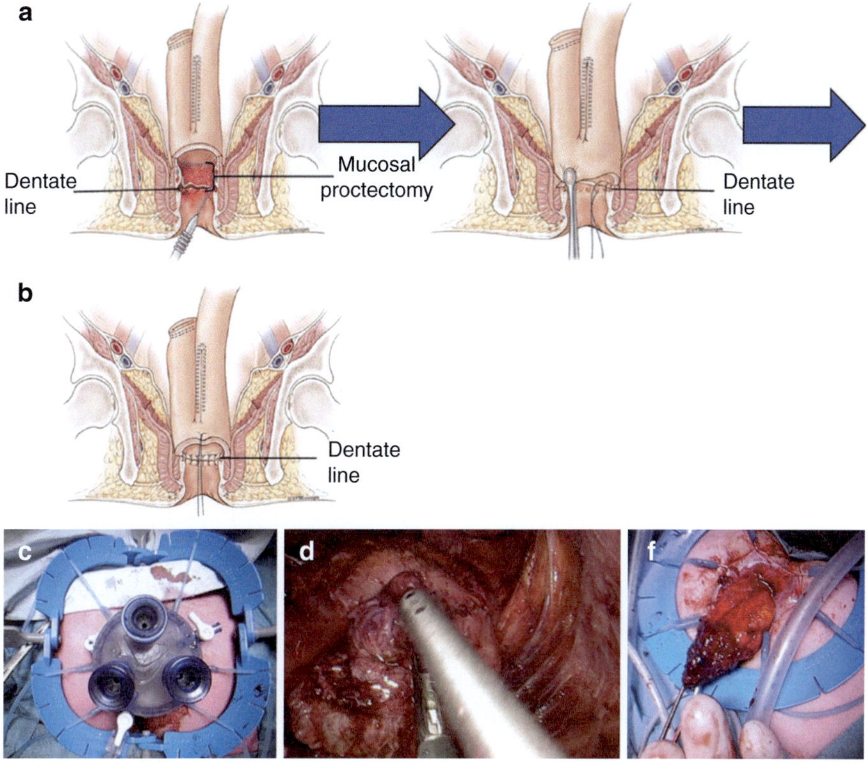


**Fig. 6.11** (**a–c**) Cuff/efferent loop excision; (**a**) incision of the rectal mucosa, (**b**) mobilization and excision of the cuff/efferent loop, (**c**) handsewn anastomosis. (**d**) TAMIS platform for transanal surgery, (**e**) TAMIS view on transanally mobilized pouch, (**f**) exteriorization of mobilized distal part of the pouch

**Retained rectum** The rectal wall is transected 2 cm cranial from the dentate line. Applying a close rectal dissection technique, the retained rectum is dissected until the ileorectal anastomosis is encountered. Thereafter, the pouch is carefully mobilized in order to preserve the pouch. Since the pouch must be brought down over a considerable distance, either laparoscopically or open (Pfannenstiehl or lower midline) mobilization of the pouch and its mesentery is necessary. After freeing the pouch including the pouch rectal anastomosis and the retained rectum, the latter two are excised. Preferably a single stapling double purse string ileoanal anastomosis is done to join the pouch with the anus. A small rim of cuff is preserved for better continence.

(b) *Transanal and trans abdominal mobilization of the pouch with revision of the pouch or new pouch in case of megapouch or chronic pelvic sepsis.*

The TAMIS platform is placed in the anal canal aand depending on the type of previous ileoanal anastomosis, the rectal cuff is transected just below the anastomosis taking care not to damage the internal sphincter. A mucosectomy and transection of the muscular wall at a higher level may be necessary. The first part of the bottom up dissection can be done using retractors or via the TAMIS platform. The bottom up TAMIS dissection is carried out as far as possible after which the rendezvous is made after top down dissection of pouch and its mesentery. The completely detached and mobilized pouch can be remodeled. In case of megapouch, the pouch must be reduced in size. Care must be taken when reducing the pouch size longitudinally, so that the vascularization of parts of the remaining pouch is not compromised. For pelvic sepsis, the pouch is often reduced in size due to the required excision of the distal part. Quite often a blind loop is present, giving the opportunity to enlarge the pouch by incorporating the blind loop into the lumen of the pouch using lineair staplers. Presacral sinuses must be carefully debrided to prevent recurrent abscesses. The ileoanal anastomosis should be handsewn using interrupted Vicryl 3-0 sutures with defunctioning as a routine. A pelvic drain is left in place for 48 h and 5 days of antibiotics are prescribed in the patients that were operated for pelvic sepsis.

(c) *Transanal and transabdominal intersphincteric excision of the pouch with omental plasty in case of pelvic sepsis or Crohn's disease of the pouch.*

The incision is made at the level of the groove between the internal and external anal sphincter muscle. The intersphincteric plane is followed up to the ileoanal anastomosis. Next, the TAMIS port is inserted and the bottom up dissection is proceeded via TAMIS. Either via low midline laparotomy or via laparoscopy the top down dissection is proceeded until the rendezvous is made. The pouch is excised and an end loop ileostomy is made. If there is sufficient omentum, a pediculised omentoplasty is performed after careful debridement of any sceptic pockets in the pelvis. If there is no omentum, a close bowel excision of the pouch can be performed in order to use the pouch mesentery to fill the pelvic cavity [22] (Fig. 6.12a, b).

(d) Transanal cleavage of pouch septa.

In the event of pouch septa, the septa can be transected using laparoscopic stapler under general anesthesia.

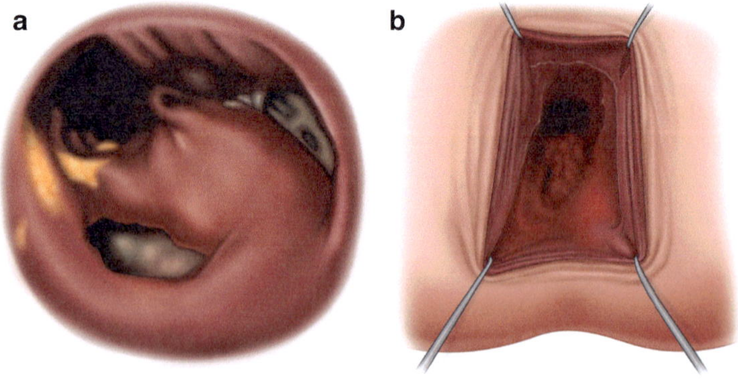


**Fig. 6.12** (**a**) J-pouch after pelvic sepsis. (**b**) Transanal view

### 6.4.2 *Results of Redo Surgery*

The largest series of pouch redo operations originates from the Cleveland Clinic Ohio. Remzi et al. described over 500 patients having redo pouch surgery over a 20 years' time period [28–31]. The main indication for pouch redo surgery were septic problems of the anastomosis (61%), emptying problems (23%) and pouch vaginal fistula (17%). Success rates were 90% at 5 years and 82% at 10 years' time. Independent factors of failure of redo surgery were septic problems as an indication for pouch revision and postoperative complications after redo surgery. Smaller series confirmed Remzi's observation that results of redo surgery were best in patients having mechanical causes of pouch dysfunction as opposed to those who have inflammatory/septic causes [32, 33]. Patients with true Crohn's disease had less favorable results. It has to be stressed that many patients with septic pouch problems are labelled as having Crohn's disease while they in fact have a complicated pouch [27].

In the systematic review of Theodoropoulos, he reported favorable results in terms of healing rates for the redo, revisional, and local/perineal pouch procedures of 82.2%, 79.6%, and 68.4%, respectively [23]. However, due to the considerably lower morbidity rate associated with the performance of a local/perineal pouch repair, as demonstrated in the review (13.6% vs 44.2% for the revisional surgery), some authors have suggested that all revisional surgery should be first attempted transanally, with the aim of local repair. Theodoropoulos reported functionally worse outcomes for urgency and night-time soiling, 26% and 38.4% respectively, compared to the reported rates of 7.3%, 17.3%, and 7.6% for urgency, mild, and severe nighttime incontinence, respectively, after initial restorative proctocolectomy. This functional deterioration might be attributable to repeated sphincter trauma, mucosectomy, handsewn anastomosis, decreased small bowel length in the patients who need to undergo redo procedures.

## References


1. Lovegrove RE, Heriot AG, Constantinides V, Tilney HS, Darzi AW, Fazio VW, et al. Meta-analysis of short-term and long-term outcomes of J, W and S ileal reservoirs for restorative proctocolectomy. Color Dis [Internet]. 2007 [cited 2017 Jul 31];9(4):310–20. Available from: http://www.ncbi.nlm.nih.gov/pubmed/17432982
2. Lovegrove RE, Constantinides VA, Heriot AG, Athanasiou T, Darzi A, Remzi FH, et al. A comparison of hand-sewn versus stapled ileal pouch anal anastomosis (IPAA) following proctocolectomy: a meta-analysis of 4183 patients. Ann Surg [Internet]. 2006 [cited 2017 Jul 31];244(1):18–26. Available from: http://www.ncbi.nlm.nih.gov/pubmed/16794385
3. Pouch Procedure & Recovery Types of Surgeries | Cleveland Clinic [Internet]. [cited 2018 Mar 6]. Available from: https://my.clevelandclinic.org/health/treatments/17379-pouch-procedure--recovery/types-of-surgeries
4. Fazio VW, Kiran RP, Remzi FH, Coffey JC, Heneghan HM, Kirat HT, et al. Ileal pouch anal anastomosis analysis of outcome and quality of life in 3707 patients. Ann Surg

[Internet]. 2013 [cited 2017 Jul 31];257:679–85. Available from: https://insights.ovid.com/pubmed?pmid=23299522
5. Remzi FH, Fazio VW, Delaney CP, Preen M, Ormsby A, Bast J, et al. Dysplasia of the anal transitional zone after ileal pouch-anal anastomosis: results of prospective evaluation after a minimum of ten years. Dis Colon Rectum [Internet]. 2003 [cited 2017 Jul 31];46(1):6–13. Available from: http://www.ncbi.nlm.nih.gov/pubmed/12544515
6. Kirat HT, Remzi FH, Kiran RP, Fazio VW. Comparison of outcomes after hand-sewn versus stapled ileal pouch-anal anastomosis in 3,109 patients. Surgery [Internet]. 2009 [cited 2017 Aug 2];146(4):723-9-30. Available from: http://linkinghub.elsevier.com/retrieve/pii/S0039606009004577
7. Sahami S, Bartels SAL, D'Hoore A, Fadok TY, Tanis PJ, Lindeboom R, et al. A multicentre evaluation of risk factors for anastomotic leakage after restorative proctocolectomy with ileal pouch-anal anastomosis for inflammatory bowel disease. J Crohns Colitis [Internet]. 2016 [cited 2017 Jul 31];10(7):773–8. Available from: https://academic.oup.com/ecco-jcc/article-lookup/doi/10.1093/ecco-jcc/jjv170
8. Sahami S, Buskens CJ, Fadok TY, Tanis PJ, de Buck van Overstraeten A, Wolthuis AM, et al. Defunctioning ileostomy is not associated with reduced leakage in proctocolectomy and ileal pouch anastomosis surgeries for IBD. J Crohn's Colitis [Internet]. 2016 [cited 2017 Jul 31];10(7):779–85. Available from: http://www.ncbi.nlm.nih.gov/pubmed/26512136
9. Zittan E, Wong-Chong N, Ma GW, McLeod RS, Silverberg MS, Cohen Z. Modified two-stage ileal pouch-anal anastomosis results in lower rate of anastomotic leak compared with traditional two-stage surgery for ulcerative colitis. J Crohns Colitis [Internet]. 2016 [cited 2017 Jul 31];10(7):766–72. Available from: https://academic.oup.com/ecco-jcc/article-lookup/doi/10.1093/ecco-jcc/jjw069
10. Bartels SAL, D'Hoore A, Cuesta MA, Bensdorp AJ, Lucas C, Bemelman WA. Significantly increased pregnancy rates after laparoscopic restorative proctocolectomy. Ann Surg [Internet]. 2012 [cited 2017 Jul 31];256(6):1045–8. Available from: http://www.ncbi.nlm.nih.gov/pubmed/22609840
11. Bartels SAL, Gardenbroek TJ, Aarts M, Ponsioen CY, Tanis PJ, Buskens CJ, et al. Short-term morbidity and quality of life from a randomized clinical trial of close rectal dissection and total mesorectal excision in ileal pouch-anal anastomosis. Br J Surg [Internet]. 2015 [cited 2017 Jun 30];102(3):281–7. Available from: http://doi.wiley.com/10.1002/bjs.9701
12. Rink AD, Radinski I, Vestweber K-H. Does mesorectal preservation protect the ileoanal anastomosis after restorative proctocolectomy? J Gastrointest Surg [Internet]. 2009 [cited 2017 Aug 1];13(1):120–8. Available from: http://link.springer.com/10.1007/s11605-008-0665-x
13. Ito M, Sugito M, Kobayashi A, Nishizawa Y, Tsunoda Y, Saito N. Relationship between multiple numbers of stapler firings during rectal division and anastomotic leakage after laparoscopic rectal resection. Int J Color Dis [Internet]. 2008 [cited 2017 Aug 1];23(7):703–7. Available from: http://link.springer.com/10.1007/s00384-008-0470-8
14. Øresland T, Bemelman W, Sampietro G, Spinelli A, Windsor A, Tiret E, et al. European evidence based consensus on surgery for ulcerative colitis. J Crohn's Colitis [Internet]. Oxford University Press; 2014 [cited 2017 Jul 31];52(7):198–204. Available from: https://academic.oup.com/ecco-jcc/article-lookup/doi/10.1016/j.crohns.2014.08.012
15. Hueting WE, Buskens E, van der Tweel I, Gooszen HG, van Laarhoven CJHM. Results and complications after ileal pouch anal anastomosis: a meta-analysis of 43 observational studies comprising 9,317 patients. Dig Surg [Internet]. 2005 [cited 2017 Aug 1];22(1–2):69–79. Available from: http://www.karger.com/?doi=10.1159/000085356
16. Tekkis PP, Lovegrove RE, Tilney HS, Smith JJ, Sagar PM, Shorthouse AJ, et al. Long-term failure and function after restorative proctocolectomy – a multi-centre study of patients from the UK National Ileal Pouch Registry. Color Dis [Internet]. 2010 [cited 2017 Aug 1];12(5):433–41. Available from: http://doi.wiley.com/10.1111/j.1463-1318.2009.01816.x
17. Kiely JM, Fazio VW, Remzi FH, Shen B, Kiran RP. Pelvic sepsis after IPAA adversely affects function of the pouch and quality of life. Dis Colon Rectum [Internet]. 2012 [cited 2017 Aug

1];55(4):387–92. Available from: http://content.wkhealth.com/linkback/openurl?sid=WKPTLP:landingpage&an=00003453-201204000-00004
18. Selvaggi F, Sciaudone G, Limongelli P, Di Stazio C, Guadagni I, Pellino G, et al. The effect of pelvic septic complications on function and quality of life after ileal pouch-anal anastomosis: a single center experience. Am Surg [Internet]. 2010 [cited 2017 Aug 1];76(4):428–35. Available from: http://www.ncbi.nlm.nih.gov/pubmed/20420256
19. Weidenhagen R, Gruetzner KU, Wiecken T, Spelsberg F, Jauch K-W. Endoscopic vacuum-assisted closure of anastomotic leakage following anterior resection of the rectum: a new method. Surg Endosc [Internet]. 2008 [cited 2017 Aug 1];22(8):1818–25. Available from: http://www.ncbi.nlm.nih.gov/pubmed/18095024
20. Gardenbroek TJ, Musters GD, Buskens CJ, Ponsioen CY, D'Haens GRAM, Dijkgraaf MGW, et al. Early reconstruction of the leaking ileal pouch-anal anastomosis: a novel solution to an old problem. Color Dis [Internet]. 2015 [cited 2017 Aug 1];17(5):426–32. Available from: http://doi.wiley.com/10.1111/codi.12867
21. Liska D, Mino J. When "pouchitis" isn't pouchitis: Crohn's disease and surgical complications. Semin Colon Rectal Surg [Internet]. W.B. Saunders; 2017 [cited 2018 Mar 6];28(3):142–9. Available from: https://www.sciencedirect.com/science/article/pii/S1043148917300453
22. Joyce MR, Fazio VW, Hull TT, Church J, Kiran RP, Mor I, et al. Ileal pouch prolapse: prevalence, management, and outcomes. J Gastrointest Surg [Internet]. 2010 [cited 2017 Aug 1];14(6):993–7. Available from: http://link.springer.com/10.1007/s11605-010-1194-y
23. Ehsan M, Isler JT, Kimmins MH, Billingham RP. Prevalence and management of prolapse of the ileoanal pouch. Dis Colon Rectum [Internet]. 2004 [cited 2017 Aug 1];47(6):885–8. Available from: http://www.ncbi.nlm.nih.gov/pubmed/15054682
24. de Groof EJ, van Ruler O, Buskens CJ, Tanis PJ, Bemelman WA. Mesenteric tissue for the treatment of septic pelvic complications in the absence of greater omentum. Tech Coloproctol [Internet]. 2016 [cited 2017 Aug 1];20(12):875–8. Available from: http://www.ncbi.nlm.nih.gov/pubmed/27909892
25. Theodoropoulos GE, Choman EN, Wexner SD. Salvage procedures after restorative proctocolectomy: a systematic review and meta-analysis. J Am Coll Surg [Internet]. 2015 [cited 2017 Aug 1];220(2):225–42.e1. Available from: http://www.ncbi.nlm.nih.gov/pubmed/25535169
26. Mallick IH, Hull TL, Remzi FH, Kiran RP. Management and outcome of pouch-vaginal fistulas after IPAA surgery. Dis Colon Rectum [Internet]. 2014 [cited 2017 Aug 1];57(4):490–6. Available from: http://content.wkhealth.com/linkback/openurl?sid=WKPTLP:landingpage&an=00003453-201404000-00012
27. Litzendorf ME, Stucchi AF, Wishnia S, Lightner A, Becker JM. Completion mucosectomy for retained rectal mucosa following restorative proctocolectomy with double-stapled ileal pouch-anal anastomosis. J Gastrointest Surg [Internet]. 2010 [cited 2017 Aug 1];14(3):562–9. Available from: http://link.springer.com/10.1007/s11605-009-1099-9
28. Borstlap WAA, Harran N, Tanis PJ, Bemelman WA. Feasibility of the TAMIS technique for redo pelvic surgery. Surg Endosc [Internet]. 2016 [cited 2017 Aug 1];30(12):5364–71. Available from: http://link.springer.com/10.1007/s00464-016-4889-7
29. Garrett KA, Remzi FH, Kirat HT, Fazio VW, Shen B, Kiran RP. Outcome of salvage surgery for ileal pouches referred with a diagnosis of crohn's disease. Dis Colon Rectum [Internet]. 2009 [cited 2017 Aug 1];52(12):1967–74. Available from: http://www.ncbi.nlm.nih.gov/pubmed/19934917
30. Remzi FH, Aytac E, Ashburn J, Gu J, Hull TL, Dietz DW, et al. Transabdominal redo ileal pouch surgery for failed restorative proctocolectomy. Ann Surg [Internet]. 2015 [cited 2017 Aug 1];262(4):675–82. Available from: http://www.ncbi.nlm.nih.gov/pubmed/26366548
31. Mathis KL, Dozois EJ, Larson DW, Cima RR, Wolff BG, Pemberton JH. Outcomes in patients with ulcerative colitis undergoing partial or complete reconstructive surgery for failing ileal pouch-anal anastomosis. Ann Surg [Internet]. 2009 [cited 2017 Aug 1];249(3):409–13. Available from: http://www.ncbi.nlm.nih.gov/pubmed/19247027

32. Pellino G, Selvaggi F. Outcomes of salvage surgery for ileal pouch complications and dysfunctions. The experience of a referral centre and review of literature. J Crohns Colitis [Internet]. 2015 [cited 2017 Aug 2];9(7):548–57. Available from: https://academic.oup.com/ecco-jcc/article-lookup/doi/10.1093/ecco-jcc/jjv066
33. Heuschen UA, Allemeyer EH, Hinz U, Lucas M, Herfarth C, Heuschen G. Outcome after septic complications in J pouch procedures. Br J Surg [Internet]. 2002 [cited 2017 Aug 2];89(2):194–200. Available from: http://doi.wiley.com/10.1046/j.0007-1323.2001.01983.x

# Chapter 7
# Ileal Pouch Salvage, Pouch Failure and Redo Surgery

**Constantinos Simillis and Omar Faiz**

**Abstract** Rates of pouch failure can vary between 3.5% and 17% in the described literature. The most common causes for failure are sepsis, poor function and sepsis. In some situations revisional surgery is required and this chapter aims to describe the causation of pouch failure, revisional surgery and the functional outcomes of revisional surgery.

**Keywords** Pouch failure · Complication management · Pouch salvage · Redo surgery · Revisional surgery · Patient satisfaction · Permanent ileostomy · Quality of life

## 7.1 Indications

The main reasons for restorative proctocolectomy are for refractory ulcerative colitis or familial adenomatous polyposis [1, 2]. A conventional proctocolectomy gives excellent results, and the only reason for restorative proctocolectomy is to avoid a permanent ileostomy by restoring intestinal continuity and allowing per anal defecation. To make an informed decision, the patient should be aware of the risks of an ileal pouch-anal anastomosis, including complication and failure rates, total treatment time and understand the likely functional outcome. In most patients, restorative proctocolectomy results in acceptable function outcomes and good quality of life, but fails in between 3.5% and 17% of patients over the longer term [1–9].

C. Simillis
Department of Colorectal Surgery, West Middlesex University Hospital, Chelsea and Westminster Hospital NHS Trust, London, UK
e-mail: constantinos.simillis@chelwest.nhs.uk

O. Faiz (✉)
St. Mark's Academic Institute, Surgical Epidemiological Trials and Outcomes Centre, London, UK
e-mail: omar.faiz@nhs.net



J. Warusavitarne, Z. Perry-Woodford (eds.), *The Ileoanal Pouch*,
https://doi.org/10.1007/978-3-319-94385-5_7

The predominant causes of pouch failure are pelvic sepsis in approximately 50% of patients, poor function in 30%, and pouchitis in 10% [10]. The overall rate of pouch failure increases steadily with time following restorative proctocolectomy [10, 11]. Patients who developed pelvic sepsis in the immediate postoperative period after primary restorative proctocolectomy have a significantly higher risk of pouch failure [12–14]. Pouchitis is the most common medical complication after ileal pouch-anal anastomosis, affecting up to 50% of patients at some point, and it is more common in ulcerative colitis than in familial adenomatous polyposis patients [15, 16]. A diagnosis of pouchitis should be made based on symptoms (increased stool frequency, urgency, tenesmus, incontinence, nocturnal seepage, abdominal pain, pyrexia, dehydration, malaise, malnutrition), endoscopic and histologic findings. Surgery for pouchitis is necessary only rarely and should be considered only in cases in which there is a total lack of response to medical therapy.

In patients with pouch failure due to complications following primary ileal pouch-anal anastomosis or due to poor function, repeat pouch salvage surgery can be considered. This is usually the patients' only option to avoid a permanent stoma, and has good results for selected patients in experienced hands. The first step is to identify the cause for the pouch failure, using all the diagnostic tools available followed by a multidisciplinary evaluation. Having made a diagnosis, nonsurgical treatment is usually attempted and exhausted before surgery is considered [17]. Because pouch salvage surgery is a major undertaking and pouch salvage procedures are demanding and complicated procedures, the results are critically dependent on experience and technical proficiency. Pouch salvage surgery should be performed in specialised surgical centres which have accumulated substantial experience in performing such operations.

It is essential that patients undergoing pouch salvage surgery are supported and well informed, especially for a patient who is highly motivated to avoid a permanent ileostomy and has already suffered the disappointment and prolonged ill health due to the pouch failure after primary restorative proctocolectomy. Redo pouch surgery should be avoided in patients with poor anal sphincter function, active anal or small bowel Crohn's disease, or patients with loss of a critical amount of terminal ileum. The patient should be informed of the duration of treatment and hospital stay, the complications of surgery that may occur, and the chance of success of salvage surgery. A pouch support nurse, stoma therapist and patient-support group can offer valuable advice to the patient during this process. The patient should be aware of the risk that an end-ileostomy may be the only option once the original pouch is mobilized or resected, because the remaining small bowel may not reach to form a new pouch. Also, the patient should be warned that if a new pouch is made, the function may be worse [17, 18]. Should the salvage pouch fail the patient is likely to experience significant deterioration in quality of life as the upstream ileostomy of the redo pouch is likely to be considerably proximal to the location of the original ileocaecal valve.

There are several circumstances in which a salvage procedure is necessary to resolve a complication and to prevent pouch failure. Pouch salvage surgery aims to preserve the pouch and transanal defaecation. A recent meta-analysis by Theodoropoulos et al., identified the following indications for salvage surgery [18]:

- Sepsis (54.5%): pelvic sepsis/abscess, anastomotic leak/separation, pouch-vaginal fistula, peri-pouch fistula/sinus other than pouch-vaginal fistula
- Mechanical (44.6%): ileal pouch-anal anastomosis stenosis, poor emptying, long efferent limb, retained rectum, ischaemic pouch, pouch prolapse, straight ileal pouch-anal anastomosis, small-volume reservoir, afferent limb obstruction, pouch septum, twisted pouch, sphincter dysfunction/incontinence
- Inflammatory (0.4%)
- Neoplastic (0.3%)

Table 7.1 demonstrates the operative indications for redo ileal pouch surgery in 502 patients reported by Remzi et al. [17].

Stapling of the ileal pouch-anal anastomosis with sparing of the anal transitional zone raises concerns about the potential risk of dysplasia and adenocarcinoma in the anal transitional zone. Dysplasia is reported to occur in 2.8% of patients with a pouch [19]. The risk of carcinoma is reported to be 0.02% in patients with ulcerative colitis and 0.9% in familial adenomatous polyposis [20]. A systematic review of the literature by Selvaggi et al. to identify pouch-related adenocarcinoma in patients post restorative proctocolectomy for ulcerative colitis found a cumulative incidence of pouch-related adenocarcinoma of 0.33% 50 years after the diagnosis of ulcerative colitis and 0.35% 20 years after an ileal pouch-anal anastomosis [20]. Neoplasia on the colectomy specimen was the strongest risk factor (odds ratio, 8.8; 95% confidence interval [CI], 4.61–16.80), and mucosectomy did not abolish the risk of subsequent cancer but avoiding it increased eight times the risk of cancer arising from the residual anorectal mucosa (odds ratio, 8; 95% CI, 1.3–48.7) [20].

The indication for pouch salvage surgery after restorative proctocolectomy influences the outcome. Sepsis is the most common indication for pouch salvage surgery [11, 18], and studies have demonstrated that the outcome of salvage surgery for patients with sepsis as an indication is worse than that for patients without sepsis [11, 15, 18, 21, 22]. Whether sepsis should be considered a suitable indication for

**Table 7.1** Operative indications for redo ileal pouch surgery in 502 patients reported by Remzi and co-workers [17]

| Operative indication | Number of patients (%) |
|---|---|
| Leak/fistula | 263 (52) |
| Pouch vaginal fistula | 85 (17) |
| Obstruction | 116 (23) |
| Dysfunction | 45 (10) |
| Pelvic perianal abscess | 43 (9) |
| Pouchitis | 14 (3) |
| Prolapse | 11 (2) |
| Neoplastic | 10 (2) |

abdominal salvage is controversial [23]. Within the category of sepsis, patients with pelvic sepsis appeared to have worse outcomes than those with fistulation [11]. Approximately 3%–15% of female patients with a pouch may develop a pouch-vaginal fistula [15, 24–26] and symptoms consist of faecal discharge or gas emission through the vagina. In a study by Heriot et al. [27] including 68 patients with pouch-vaginal fistulas, the origin of the vaginal fistulas was the pouch-anal anastomosis in 52 (76.5%) patients, pouch body/top in 9 (13.2%), or cryptoglandular or other source in 7 (10.3%). The diagnosis of Crohn's disease was made in eight (12%) patients [27].

Good results have been reported with salvage surgery for the treatment of evacuation difficulty or poor pouch function [11, 15, 23, 28–31]. Tekkis et al. demonstrated that the most promising indication for successful abdominal salvage surgery is mechanical outflow obstruction at the ileoanal level, and recognised three clinicopathological conditions within this category where salvage surgery was found to have a success rate of over 80% in each of the three groups [11]:

- Obstruction caused by the distal ileal segment of an S reservoir. S pouch is however now rarely used and salvage surgery for this indication is rarely needed.
- Stenosis of the ileoanal anastomosis.
- Inadequate removal of the rectum resulting in a pouch–rectal rather than pouch–anal anastomosis. A retained rectal stump of varying length is more likely when a stapled ileal pouch-anal anastomosis is performed, but an inadequate hand-sewn technique may also be responsible for this complication. Also, laparoscopically performed pouches are often considered to have longer rectal stumps than those performed open due to the technical difficulty associated with rectal cross-stapling with minimal access techniques [17]. A retained rectal stump may lead to persisting symptoms of inflammation of the residual rectal mucosa (cuffitis) and outflow obstruction leading to an evacuation disorder that may ultimately require salvage surgery [11].

## 7.2 Surgery

When pouch failure develops, the surgical options are either to attempt a pouch salvage procedure or convert to a permanent ileostomy. If pouch excision with a permanent end-ileostomy is performed, management of the anal canal remnant is determined by reasons for pouch failure, the state of the perineum and sphincter mechanism, and the presence or absence of associated sepsis. One option is to proceed with repeat abdominal surgery, pouch resection, and abdominoperineal pouch excision and reconstruction. In some circumstances, the conversion of a J-pouch into a continent ileostomy (K-pouch) may be considered for the preservation of continence and improvement of quality of life. Alternatively, provided symptoms from the retained pouch are not unmanageable and do not impinge on quality of life, an ileostomy can be formed above a pouch left in situ. It is the authors preference to construct an end ileostomy leaving the stapled distal limb under the skin to prevent overflow of intestinal content into the distal limb and pouch. When the pouch is left in situ, it is necessary to perform periodic surveillance of the pouch with surveillance biopsies.

Pouch salvage surgery can maintain the old pouch through the application of revisional salvage procedures, and, if this is not feasible, to substitute it with a new one. Depending on the pouch complication, a variety of pouch salvage techniques have been used [9, 16, 26, 32, 33]. No definitive evidence exists on which treatment strategy is the most appropriate, and surgical treatment can be tailored to suit clinical manifestations and be individualized to optimize outcomes. Certainly, the approach under these circumstances is pragmatic. Failure of one salvage attempt should not be considered a contraindication to additional attempts. In conjunction with appropriate patient selection, surgical judgment, and individual surgeon experience, the decision as to which technical approach to use is problem specific and is largely influenced by the indication for salvage surgery [18, 34, 35]. Preoperatively the patient is assessed with a comprehensive history and physical exam, and investigations are arranged such as pouchography, pelvic MRI, CT scan of the abdomen and pelvis, anal manometry, examination under anaesthesia, and possible consultation with our gastroenterology colleagues.

In a meta-analysis by Theodoropoulos et al., the following subtypes of pouch salvage procedures have been identified [18]:

- Redo (11.3%): necessitating abdominal exploration, excision of the existing pouch and formation of a new pouch of any configuration with creation of an ileal pouch-anal anastomosis.
- Revisional (45.4%): abdominal exploration, pouch revision and correction of the pouch structural abnormality, including excision or oversewing of fistulas and/or pouch reduction or augmentation, with or without abdomino-anal advancement, and with or without disconnection of the old anastomosis and creation of a new one.
- Local/perineal (43.3%): any procedures that do not require entrance into the abdominal cavity and can be completed via the perineal, transanal, transvaginal, or transgluteal route by operative, endoscopic, or imaging-guided means [18]. Increasingly the perineal approach is being used by surgeons employing minimal access techniques to revise pouches.

In a study by Remzi et al. including 502 patients, a new pouch was created in 41% of patients whereas 59% had their original pouch revised and retained [17].

A local/perineal salvage procedure should be considered first due to its associated lower morbidity rate compared to redo or revisional procedures [18, 36]. Nevertheless, a local/perineal approach may not be adequate for the correction of the responsible pathology, and the rate of reoperations to achieve the desirable outcomes, is higher than after revisional or redo surgery [18]. Patients that need a redo or revisional salvage surgery are offered a three-stage procedure. The first stage would be an end stoma (derived from a diverting loop ileostomy with the distal limb stapled under the surface), which detoxifies the patient and reconditions them [17].

It allows the patient to feel better, prepare mentally, optimize their nutrition, gain weight, and improve physically overall in order to achieve the best possible outcome with salvage surgery. It also enables them to revisit life with a stoma. This is followed by a redo or revisional surgery after 6 months. Then ileostomy closure would be scheduled approximately 3 months after redo or revisional surgery. Examination under anaesthesia, pouchoscopy, gastrograffin enema, and possible pelvic MRI are used to confirm pouch and anastomotic integrity, without any leaks and/or obstruction, before proceeding with ileostomy closure. If any complication is noticed, ileostomy reversal is delayed and the complication treated.

During redo or revisional pouch surgery the patient is placed in the Lloyd-Davies position, and both the abdomen and perineum are prepared and draped for surgery. Bilateral ureteric stents are placed in most patients to allow the identification of the ureters and detection of any injury. The previous incision is used for laparotomy or a midline incision is made for those previously operated by the laparoscopic technique. A thorough exploration of the abdomen is performed, and the entire small bowel is cautiously mobilized. The small bowel mesentery and pouch are mobilised down to the level of the pelvic floor and levators with sharp dissection, ensuring preservation of the presacral nerves and other pelvic structures. If the salvage surgery is performed because of pouch failure resulting from a chronic presacral abscess cavity, the abscess is drained and the cavity wall is debrided.

The pouch can be disconnected from the anastomosis, delivered into the abdomen, evaluated, inspected for structural defects, and measured. At this stage, the decision is made on whether to excise the old pouch and create a new one, or to repair/revise/reattach the old pouch. This decision is based on the viability and integrity of the existing pouch after complete mobilization, its residual capacity, the length of the remaining small intestine, the ability of the new pouch to reach the anus without excess tension, and the cause of pouch failure. Repair of the old pouch generally requires mobilization and disconnection from the anus, with a redo anastomosis. An important reason for retaining the old pouch, if possible, is preservation of the small bowel, especially the critical last 60 cm [17]. In the case of redo pouch surgery, the pre-pouch neo-terminal ileum is used to create the new pouch. Most commonly a repeat handsewn ileal pouch-anal anastomosis is performed after mucosectomy to the level of the dentate line. In certain circumstances, where a long rectal cuff has been retained a double purse string anastomosis may be feasible. The pouch is pulled through the pelvis and anastomosed with a series of interrupted sutures. A routine loop ileostomy is advised, as it minimizes the effects of a possible leak.

The integral components of revisional surgery for pelvic sepsis are repair of any pouch or anastomotic defects, excision of the phlegmon, and removal of sepsis-related fibrotic and necrotic pelvic tissues, and abdomino-anal advancement of the preserved pouch [11, 18, 34–37]. Otherwise, a redo salvage procedure can be performed, or the pouch is resected and a permanent end-ileostomy is formed. In a limited number of patients antibiotics can be used to treat pelvic sepsis, or there is spontaneous drainage of the sepsis through the ileal pouch-anal anastomosis. Also, peri-pouch abscesses can be drained through the pouch–anal anastomosis under anaesthesia or a CT-guided drainage can be performed. In cases of chronic, posterior (presacral) sinuses originating from the ileal pouch-anal anastomosis the use of repeated application of endosponges in the sinus from the anastomosis can be attempted [38], (see chapter by Bemelman) or otherwise, abdominoperineal salvage surgery can be performed with pouch disconnection and debridement and redo of the ileal pouch-anal anastomosis [15, 39]. Most of the techniques described above to treat pelvic sepsis only relate to the early postoperative period. Long standing pelvic sepsis leads to induration.

In cases of sepsis related to a fistula, especially pouch-vaginal fistula, repairs like plain fistulectomy do not offer definitive cure and seton placement can be used temporarily for control of sepsis only [25, 32, 40, 41]. For pouch-vaginal fistulas originating above the ileal pouch-anal anastomosis, or if there is a significant length of anorectal stump below the level of the fistula, an abdominal approach is required and pouch revision or redo salvage surgery is performed, with primary repair of the vaginal defect, resection of the potentially retained rectum, mucosectomy, and advancement of the ileal pouch-anal anastomosis below the level of the fistula [27]. For pouch-vaginal fistulas originating below the ileal pouch-anal anastomosis, local procedures can be attempted first and include transanal or transvaginal advancement full-thickness flap repair. Endoanal flap advancements are technically difficult in patients with stapled anastomosis, whereas transvaginal repair allows direct access to the fistula avoiding potential sphincter damage [18, 34].

Stricture of the ileal pouch-anal anastomosis causing outflow obstruction can be treated with repeated dilation using Hegar dilators under anaesthesia [21]. Short stenoses, up to 2 cm in length, can be managed by transanal posterior strictureplasty. Patients not responding to treatment, or with long fibrotic strictures, require an abdominoperineal approach which includes disconnection of the ileal pouch-anal anastomosis, removal of the fibrotic ring and redo of the anastomosis [15, 42]. Similarly, in the presence of cuffitis, a transanal mucosectomy may control symptoms, or a transanal ileal pouch-anal anastomosis disconnection with anastomosis advancement can be performed, but in unresponsive patients a combined abdominoperineal approach is required, with abdominal mobilization of the pouch, removal of the retained rectal stump and transanal mucosectomy with redo ileal pouch-anal anastomosis [11].

In patients with a long efferent pouch limb (e.g. after S pouch) causing outlet obstruction and requiring intermittent catheterisation, the long efferent limb can be removed transanally by mobilizing the pouch, disconnecting the ileal pouch-anal anastomosis, and excising the long efferent pouch limb. In cases of afferent limb syndrome where small-bowel obstruction is caused by acute angulation, prolapse or intussusception of the afferent limb at the junction to the pouch, surgical options include resection of the angulated bowel, pouchopexy, mobilization with fixation of the small bowel, and pouch excision [15, 43].

Pouch prolapse, defined as a protrusion of the pouch through the anus, can be managed surgically through a transanal excision of the prolapsed mucosa, or through an abdominoperineal salvage approach with pouchopexy for full-thickness pouch prolapse [44, 45].

Twists in the pouch mesentery or pouch volvulus can occur, especially after laparoscopic pouch formation, and an emergency laparotomy is required with untwisting of the pouch, and pouchopexy or pouch excision [46, 47]. The likelihood of a mesenteric twist can be minimized by making sure that the cut edge of the small bowel mesentery is straight and passes up and to the right toward the stump of the ileocolic artery [17].

There is an inverse relationship between the capacity of the reservoir and bowel frequency [48], and inadequate pouch volume may be responsible for pouch malfunction. For a small-volume reservoir, abdominal pouch salvage with pouch enhancement can reduce bowel frequency and rescue the pouch [15, 36]. Small pouch reservoirs can be enlarged by approximating one or two cranial loops, opening the pouch, and suturing these to the pouch body. Poorly functioning ileal reservoirs secondary to a limited capacity and compliance can be managed with conversion to a W pouch which results in increased pouch capacity, improvement in compliance and decreased frequency of defecation [49, 50]. On the other hand, excessive pouch enlargement, due to formation of a large reservoir, can lead to dysfunction because of incomplete emptying [46]. In such cases, the volume of large pouches can be reduced by stapling reduction of a proximal portion of the pouch [46].

In cases of low-grade dysplasia arising from the residual anorectal mucosa after stapled ileal pouch-anal anastomosis or inadequate mucosectomy, the options are a wait-and-see approach with regular surveillance or mucosectomy with advancement of the anastomosis [51]. In cases of high-grade dysplasia most surgeons proceed with pouch excision, especially if there is an associated mass [20, 51]. Pouch excision should be performed in the presence of carcinoma. Although there is no consensus regarding the role of neoadjuvant or adjuvant chemotherapy or radiotherapy [20, 51] the high rate of positive resection margins in this context makes neo-adjuvant treatment approaches sensible.

## 7.3 Outcomes

MacLean et al., reported a mean operative time for pouch salvage surgery of 4 h (+/−1.1), average blood loss of 500 mL (+/−400), and average length of stay of 10.3 days (+/−4.6) [34]. Remzi et al., reported a median operating time of 246 min (range: 29–720 min), and median intraoperative blood loss of 300 mL (range: 20–2000 mL) [17]. Out of the 502 patients included in the study, there were three intraoperative ureteric injuries [17]. In the same study, median length of stay after surgery was 7 days (range: 3–57 days) and the readmission rate was 13% [17]. The morbidity rate after pouch salvage surgery is in proximity to the reported morbidity rates after primary ileal pouch-anal anastomosis. The meta-analysis by Theodoropoulos et al. reported an overall morbidity rate of 41.4% (95% CI, 21.7–61.2%) after pouch salvage surgery. The most common complications observed were pouch fistula (15.2%), stricture (13.5%), pelvic abscess (10%), pouchitis (9.2%), wound infection (9.2%), small bowel obstruction (8.3%) and pouch-vaginal

**Table 7.2** Short-term complications after redo ileal pouch surgery in 502 patients reported by Remzi and co-workers [17]

| Complications | Number of patients (%) |
|---|---|
| Pelvic sepsis | 50 (10) |
| Ileus/bowel obstruction | 81 (16) |
| Anastomotic leak | 38 (8) |
| Wound infection | 41 (8) |
| Urinary | 25 (5) |
| Cardiopulmonary | 21 (4) |
| Haemorrhage | 13 (3) |
| Anastomotic stricture | 13 (3) |
| Fistula | 13 (3) |
| Venous thromboembolism | 12 (2) |
| Pouchitis | 8 (2) |
| Stoma complications | 6 (1) |
| Bowel perforation | 2 (0.4) |
| Wound dehiscence | 2 (0.4) |

fistula (6.9%) [18]. Remzi et al., reported a postoperative mortality of 0%, morbidity of 53%, and the short-term anastomotic leak rate was 8% [17]. Table 7.2 demonstrates the short-term complications after redo ileal pouch surgery in 502 patients reported by Remzi et al. [17].

MacLean et al., reported that complications were more frequent in those who had pouch excision with creation of a new pouch (redo salvage surgery) compared with those whose old pouch was used (revisional salvage surgery) [34]. Theodoropoulos et al., reported higher frequency of complications post revisional salvage surgery (44.2%; 95% CI, 13.6–74.7%) compared with local/perineal salvage procedures (13.6%; 95% CI, 0–66.1%) [18]. In addition, the rate of postoperative complications was higher in patients who had a septic indication for salvage surgery compared with those who had an outlet problem [34].

Rates of success, defined by the avoidance of a permanent ileostomy with preservation of anal function, range from 50% to 95%, with 'good' functional results reported in 48–93% of patients [11, 18, 23, 28, 29, 34, 36, 52, 53]. A meta-analysis by Theodoropoulos et al., demonstrated overall successful healing rates after salvage surgery of 73.5% (95% CI, 67.5–79.5%) [18], and specifically, the healing success rates based on the subtype of salvage procedures performed were 82.2% (95% CI, 72.5–91.9%) for redo salvage procedures, 79.6% (95% CI, 75.7–83.5%) for revisional, and 68.4% (95% CI, 57.5–79.3%) for local/perineal salvage procedures [18]. Figure 7.1 shows a proposed algorithm published by Theodoropoulos et al. [18] for managing pouch complications and relative success rates of the various salvage options.

The indication for salvage surgery influences outcome, and studies suggested that a successful result after abdominal salvage was more likely for patients with a non-septic indication compared with those with sepsis [11, 21, 22]. Heuschen et al. reported an overall failure rate following salvage surgery of 31% at 5 years in a patient group of 131 patients with sepsis [13]. Failure was more common when

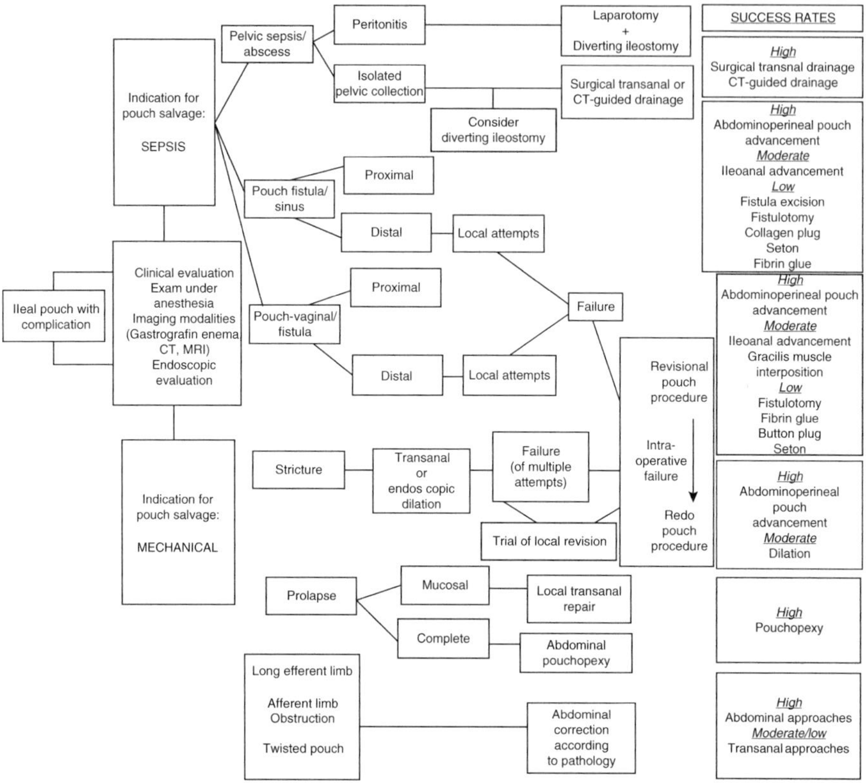


**Fig. 7.1** Proposed algorithm for managing pouch complications and relative success rates of the various salvage options published by Theodoropoulos et al. [18]

sepsis involved the lower pelvis [13]. In the recent study by Remzi et al. which included 502 patients with a median follow-up of 7 years after redo surgery, 101 (20%) patients had redo failure [17]. Postoperative complication in the short-term and pelvic sepsis were independent risk factors for pouch failure after redo ileal pouch surgery [17]. A transabdominal re-redo ileal pouch-anal anastomosis was performed in 16 patients and the pouch was salvaged in 13 patients, suggesting that select patients with a failed redo pouch can be candidates for a further redo, with a good expectation of success [17].

Good results after salvage surgery have been reported for treatment of evacuation difficulty or poor pouch function [11, 28, 31]. An 80% success rate has been reported with abdominal salvage surgery for mechanical outflow obstruction at the ileoanal level [11]. In the review by Theodoropoulos et al., pouch stenosis was the predominant mechanical indication for salvage surgery and dilations were associated with highly satisfactory success rates [18]. After dilation of pouch stenosis under anaesthesia, recurrence was found to occur within 3 years in 60% of patients, and repeated dilation can be effective in more than 50% of patients [21]. Tulchinsky et al., reported on 22 patients with a retained rectal stump who underwent abdomino-anal revision with pouch mobilization, close rectal dissection and pouch revision [31]. Five patients (22.7%) had subsequent pouch excision, whereas 15 out of 17 patients with successful salvage had marked subjective improvement in pouch function and quality of life at a median follow-up of 22 months [31].

In the review by Theodoropoulos et al., the percentage of newly diagnosed Crohn's disease patients was 11.9% among those who had been initially operated on for ulcerative colitis [18]. Mathis et al. [37], identified 22 patients with Crohn's disease out of 51 patients with a previously reported history of ulcerative colitis undergoing pouch salvage surgery. The authors found that Crohn's disease and partial revision were associated with an increased risk of complications after pouch reconstruction [37]. Also, Crohn's disease is a strong determinant for failure of salvage surgery [11, 12, 27]. Pouch salvage surgery failed in all patients with Crohn's disease in a study by Tekkis et al., and a pathological diagnosis of Crohn's disease or indeterminate colitis was associated with a higher failure rate than ulcerative colitis or familial adenomatous polyposis [11]. Alternatively, one investigator Garrett et al., reported on 33 patients with Crohn's disease who underwent a redo or revisional pouch surgery by the abdominal approach (laparotomy with creation of new pouch or revision of existing pouch with redo ileal pouch-anal anastomosis) and found a pouch survival rate of 84.8% after a median follow-up of 1.7 years, and concluded that redo pouch surgery in patients with Crohn's disease is associated with good long-term outcomes [54]. The experience of most surgeons in the context of Crohn's disease contradicts this. Moreover, most clinicians would not select patients with pouch failure secondary to Crohn's for redo surgery.

For pouch-vaginal fistulas, the transabdominal salvage procedures appear to be associated with a greater chance of success (72%) and with the least probability of reintervention (15%) [18, 32]. The review by Theodoropoulos et al., reported a success rate of only 33.3% for transvaginal repair [18]. Among 136 patients with pouch-vaginal fistula reported in the review on by Lolohea et al., 50% achieved a successful outcome, whereas 25% experienced tolerable disturbances, and 25% eventually needed permanent diversion or pouch excision [26]. Heriot et al., reported an overall pouch failure rate for patients with pouch-vaginal fistulas of 35% with median pouch survival of 4.2 years [27]. They also reported that repair in those patients with Crohn's disease uniformly failed within 5 years from primary repair [27]. They concluded that patients with recurrent pouch-vaginal fistulas and ulcerative colitis should be offered salvage surgery because successful closure following initial failure occurs in approximately 50% [27]. Tsujinaka et al., suggested that faecal diversion and local procedures are effective in the majority of patients with pouch-vaginal fistula and found that pelvic sepsis is a predictive factor of poor outcome [55]. Similarly, Shah et al., observed that local repairs can be successful with good functional outcomes, and if local repairs are not possible, or have failed, redo salvage surgery may also achieve healing [40].

Tekkis et al. [11] reported pouch failure rates of 21.4% after pouch salvage surgery, based on 112 patients undergoing 117 pouch salvage procedures, with a median follow-up of 46 months. Remzi and colleagues included 241 patients with a median follow-up of 5 years and reported a pouch failure rate of 15%. The meta-analysis by

Theodoropoulos and colleagues demonstrated that among a total of 927 patients post pouch salvage surgery, 18% eventually underwent pouch excision (110 patients) or permanent diversion (57 patients) [18]. The failure rates were higher for local/perineal (21.3%; 95% CI, 11.7–31%) compared with revisional salvage procedures (15.7%; 95% CI, 10.9–20.4%) [18]. The development of a pelvic abscess was reported to be associated with pouch failure after pouch revision [37]. Tekkis et al. found a pouch survival rate at 5 years of 85% for patients undergoing reconstructive surgery for a non-septic indication, whereas the pouch survival rate was 61% in patients with sepsis [11]. The same authors also suggested that the type of pouch design or anastomosis was not related to pouch survival [11]. The pouch failure rate after salvage surgery was found to increase with length of follow-up, with reported pouch survival rate of 88–93% at 1 year and 70–89% at 5 years [11, 37].

Functional results after salvage surgery are usually inferior compared to primary restorative proctocolectomy. This functional deterioration might be attributable to repeated sphincter trauma, mucosectomy, handsewn anastomosis, decreased small bowel length in the patients who need to undergo redo procedures, and decreased compliance of a chronically inflamed pouch in patients who require a revisional salvage surgery [18, 34]. Nevertheless, studies concluded that repeat pouch surgery was associated with satisfactory functional outcomes and quality of life in most patients [37, 56]. The meta-analysis by Theodoropoulos determined functional success rates of 71.9% (95% CI, 60–83.8%) overall for salvage surgery, 83.9% (95% CI, 55.6–100%) for redo salvage procedures, 75.8% (95% CI, 69.1–82.5%) for revisional surgery, and 71% (95% CI, 40.6–100%) for local/perineal procedures [18]. The same review reported pooled rates of 26% and 38.4% for urgency and nighttime soiling respectively, which are worse than the reported rates of 7.3%, 17.3%, and 7.6% for urgency, mild, and severe nighttime incontinence, respectively, after initial restorative proctocolectomy [57, 58].

Remzi and colleagues reported daytime and nighttime stool frequencies of 6 [1–15] and 2 (0–9), respectively, and approximately 50% of patients had seepage and used pads by day and night [17]. Also, about one-third of patients had dietary restrictions, 18% of patients had social restrictions, 18% of patients had work restriction, and 22% of patients had sexual restrictions [17]. In the study by Mathis et al., patients reported 5 daytime and 1 nighttime bowel movements [37]. Also, 43% of patients had occasional and 4% had frequent daytime incontinence [37]. The latter results are broadly in keeping with patients undergoing primary restorative proctocolectomy. Pellino et al., reported a median bowel frequency of 12.1 [7–15] and 6.9 [2–11], before and after salvage surgery, and urgency was found in 60% patients preoperatively and in 24% after salvage [15]. Irrespective of the functional outcomes, the quality of life of pouch reconstruction patients were similar to that for patients who had a successful initial restorative proctocolectomy [18, 34]. Also, patient satisfaction rates after salvage surgery were reported at high levels [43, 45, 56, 59–62] and this may be related to the patients' contentment with maintaining their pouch and their strong motivation to avoid a permanent ileostomy [17, 18]. Remzi reported that more than 90% of patients would have repeat pouch surgery again if needed and would recommend surgery to other patients [17].

## References

1. Fazio VW, Ziv Y, Church JM, et al. Ileal pouch-anal anastomoses complications and function in 1005 patients. Ann Surg. 1995;222(2):120–7.
2. Setti-Carraro P, Ritchie JK, Wilkinson KH, et al. The first 10 years' experience of restorative proctocolectomy for ulcerative colitis. Gut. 1994;35(8):1070–5.
3. Belliveau P, Trudel J, Vasilevsky CA, et al. Ileoanal anastomosis with reservoirs: complications and long-term results. Can J Surg. 1999;42(5):345–52.
4. Foley EF, Schoetz DJ Jr, Roberts PL, et al. Rediversion after ileal pouch-anal anastomosis. Causes of failures and predictors of subsequent pouch salvage. Dis Colon Rectum. 1995;38(8):793–8.
5. Gemlo BT, Wong WD, Rothenberger DA, et al. Ileal pouch-anal anastomosis. Patterns of failure. Arch Surg. 1992;127(7):784–6; discussion 787.
6. Korsgen S, Keighley MR. Causes of failure and life expectancy of the ileoanal pouch. Int J Colorectal Dis. 1997;12(1):4–8.
7. MacRae HM, McLeod RS, Cohen Z, et al. Risk factors for pelvic pouch failure. Dis Colon Rectum. 1997;40(3):257–62.
8. Meagher AP, Farouk R, Dozois RR, et al. J ileal pouch-anal anastomosis for chronic ulcerative colitis: complications and long-term outcome in 1310 patients. Br J Surg. 1998;85(6):800–3.
9. Tulchinsky H, Cohen CR, Nicholls RJ. Salvage surgery after restorative proctocolectomy. Br J Surg. 2003;90(8):909–21.
10. Tulchinsky H, Hawley PR, Nicholls J. Long-term failure after restorative proctocolectomy for ulcerative colitis. Ann Surg. 2003;238(2):229–34.
11. Tekkis PP, Heriot AG, Smith JJ, et al. Long-term results of abdominal salvage surgery following restorative proctocolectomy. Br J Surg. 2006;93(2):231–7.
12. Fazio VW, Tekkis PP, Remzi F, et al. Quantification of risk for pouch failure after ileal pouch anal anastomosis surgery. Ann Surg. 2003;238(4):605–14; discussion 614-7.
13. Heuschen UA, Allemeyer EH, Hinz U, et al. Outcome after septic complications in J pouch procedures. Br J Surg. 2002;89(2):194–200.
14. Heuschen UA, Hinz U, Allemeyer EH, et al. Risk factors for ileoanal J pouch-related septic complications in ulcerative colitis and familial adenomatous polyposis. Ann Surg. 2002;235(2):207–16.
15. Pellino G, Selvaggi F. Outcomes of salvage surgery for ileal pouch complications and dysfunctions. The experience of a referral centre and review of literature. J Crohns Colitis. 2015;9(7):548–57.
16. Sagar PM, Pemberton JH. Intraoperative, postoperative and reoperative problems with ileoanal pouches. Br J Surg. 2012;99(4):454–68.
17. Remzi FH, Aytac E, Ashburn J, et al. Transabdominal redo ileal pouch surgery for failed restorative proctocolectomy: lessons learned over 500 patients. Ann Surg. 2015;262(4):675–82.
18. Theodoropoulos GE, Choman EN, Wexner SD. Salvage procedures after restorative proctocolectomy: a systematic review and meta-analysis. J Am Coll Surg. 2015;220(2):225–42. e1
19. Remzi FH, Fazio VW, Delaney CP, et al. Dysplasia of the anal transitional zone after ileal pouch-anal anastomosis: results of prospective evaluation after a minimum of ten years. Dis Colon Rectum. 2003;46(1):6–13.
20. Selvaggi F, Pellino G, Canonico S, et al. Systematic review of cuff and pouch cancer in patients with ileal pelvic pouch for ulcerative colitis. Inflamm Bowel Dis. 2014;20(7):1296–308.
21. Galandiuk S, Scott NA, Dozois RR, et al. Ileal pouch-anal anastomosis. Reoperation for pouch-related complications. Ann Surg. 1990;212(4):446–52; discussion 452-4.
22. Senapati A, Tibbs CJ, Ritchie JK, et al. Stenosis of the pouch anal anastomosis following restorative proctocolectomy. Int J Colorectal Dis. 1996;11(2):57–9.
23. Sagar PM, Dozois RR, Wolff BG, et al. Disconnection, pouch revision and reconnection of the ileal pouch-anal anastomosis. Br J Surg. 1996;83(10):1401–5.

24. Gaertner WB, Witt J, Madoff RD, et al. Ileal pouch fistulas after restorative proctocolectomy: management and outcomes. Tech Coloproctol. 2014;18(11):1061–6.
25. Keighley MR, Grobler SP. Fistula complicating restorative proctocolectomy. Br J Surg. 1993;80(8):1065–7.
26. Lolohea S, Lynch AC, Robertson GB, et al. Ileal pouch-anal anastomosis-vaginal fistula: a review. Dis Colon Rectum. 2005;48(9):1802–10.
27. Heriot AG, Tekkis PP, Smith JJ, et al. Management and outcome of pouch-vaginal fistulas following restorative proctocolectomy. Dis Colon Rectum. 2005;48(3):451–8.
28. Fonkalsrud EW, Bustorff-Silva J. Reconstruction for chronic dysfunction of ileoanal pouches. Ann Surg. 1999;229(2):197–204.
29. Herbst F, Sielezneff I, Nicholls RJ. Salvage surgery for ileal pouch outlet obstruction. Br J Surg. 1996;83(3):368–71.
30. Nicholls RJ, Gilbert JM. Surgical correction of the efferent ileal limb for disordered defaecation following restorative proctocolectomy with the S ileal reservoir. Br J Surg. 1990;77(2):152–4.
31. Tulchinsky H, McCourtney JS, Rao KV, et al. Salvage abdominal surgery in patients with a retained rectal stump after restorative proctocolectomy and stapled anastomosis. Br J Surg. 2001;88(12):1602–6.
32. Maslekar S, Sagar PM, Harji D, et al. The challenge of pouch-vaginal fistulas: a systematic review. Tech Coloproctol. 2012;16(6):405–14.
33. Ramirez RL, Fleshner P. Reoperative inflammatory bowel disease surgery. Clin Colon Rectal Surg. 2006;19(4):195–206.
34. MacLean AR, O'Connor B, Parkes R, et al. Reconstructive surgery for failed ileal pouch-anal anastomosis: a viable surgical option with acceptable results. Dis Colon Rectum. 2002;45(7):880–6.
35. Shawki S, Belizon A, Person B, et al. What are the outcomes of reoperative restorative proctocolectomy and ileal pouch-anal anastomosis surgery? Dis Colon Rectum. 2009;52(5):884–90.
36. Fazio VW, Wu JS, Lavery IC. Repeat ileal pouch-anal anastomosis to salvage septic complications of pelvic pouches: clinical outcome and quality of life assessment. Ann Surg. 1998;228(4):588–97.
37. Mathis KL, Dozois EJ, Larson DW, et al. Outcomes in patients with ulcerative colitis undergoing partial or complete reconstructive surgery for failing ileal pouch-anal anastomosis. Ann Surg. 2009;249(3):409–13.
38. Van Koperen PJ, Van Berge Henegouwen MI, Slors JF, et al. Endo-sponge treatment of anastomotic leakage after ileo-anal pouch anastomosis: report of two cases. Colorectal Dis. 2008;10(9):943–4.
39. Gorgun E, Remzi FH. Complications of ileoanal pouches. Clin Colon Rectal Surg. 2004;17(1):43–55.
40. Shah NS, Remzi F, Massmann A, et al. Management and treatment outcome of pouch-vaginal fistulas following restorative proctocolectomy. Dis Colon Rectum. 2003;46(7):911–7.
41. Wexner SD, Rothenberger DA, Jensen L, et al. Ileal pouch vaginal fistulas: incidence, etiology, and management. Dis Colon Rectum. 1989;32(6):460–5.
42. Prudhomme M, Dozois RR, Godlewski G, et al. Anal canal strictures after ileal pouch-anal anastomosis. Dis Colon Rectum. 2003;46(1):20–3.
43. Kirat HT, Remzi FH, Shen B, et al. Pelvic abscess associated with anastomotic leak in patients with ileal pouch-anal anastomosis (IPAA): transanastomotic or CT-guided drainage? Int J Colorectal Dis. 2011;26(11):1469–74.
44. Joyce MR, Fazio VW, Hull TT, et al. Ileal pouch prolapse: prevalence, management, and outcomes. J Gastrointest Surg. 2010;14(6):993–7.
45. Ogunbiyi OA, Korsgen S, Keighley MR. Pouch salvage. Long-term outcome. Dis Colon Rectum. 1997;40(5):548–52.
46. Poggioli G, Marchetti F, Selleri S, et al. Redo pouches: salvaging of failed ileal pouch-anal anastomoses. Dis Colon Rectum. 1993;36(5):492–6.
47. Warren C, O'Donnell ME, Gardiner KR, et al. Successful management of ileo-anal pouch volvulus. Colorectal Dis. 2011;13(1):106–7.

48. Nicholls RJ, Pezim ME. Restorative proctocolectomy with ileal reservoir for ulcerative colitis and familial adenomatous polyposis: a comparison of three reservoir designs. Br J Surg. 1985;72(6):470–4.
49. Klas J, Myers GA, Starling JR, et al. Physiologic evaluation and surgical management of failed ileoanal pouch. Dis Colon Rectum. 1998;41(7):854–61.
50. Lovegrove RE, Heriot AG, Constantinides V, et al. Meta-analysis of short-term and long-term outcomes of J, W and S ileal reservoirs for restorative proctocolectomy. Colorectal Dis. 2007;9(4):310–20.
51. Silva-Velazco J, Stocchi L, Wu XR, et al. Twenty-year-old stapled pouches for ulcerative colitis without evidence of rectal cancer: implications for surveillance strategy? Dis Colon Rectum. 2014;57(11):1275–81.
52. Gorfine SR, Fichera A, Harris MT, et al. Long-term results of salvage surgery for septic complications after restorative proctocolectomy: does fecal diversion improve outcome? Dis Colon Rectum. 2003;46(10):1339–44.
53. Zmora O, Efron JE, Nogueras JJ, et al. Reoperative abdominal and perineal surgery in ileoanal pouch patients. Dis Colon Rectum. 2001;44(9):1310–4.
54. Garrett KA, Remzi FH, Kirat HT, et al. Outcome of salvage surgery for ileal pouches referred with a diagnosis of Crohn's disease. Dis Colon Rectum. 2009;52(12):1967–74.
55. Tsujinaka S, Ruiz D, Wexner SD, et al. Surgical management of pouch-vaginal fistula after restorative proctocolectomy. J Am Coll Surg. 2006;202(6):912–8.
56. Remzi FH, Fazio VW, Kirat HT, et al. Repeat pouch surgery by the abdominal approach safely salvages failed ileal pelvic pouch. Dis Colon Rectum. 2009;52(2):198–204.
57. de Zeeuw S, Ahmed Ali U, Donders RA, et al. Update of complications and functional outcome of the ileo-pouch anal anastomosis: overview of evidence and meta-analysis of 96 observational studies. Int J Colorectal Dis. 2012;27(7):843–53.
58. Hueting WE, Buskens E, van der Tweel I, et al. Results and complications after ileal pouch anal anastomosis: a meta-analysis of 43 observational studies comprising 9,317 patients. Dig Surg. 2005;22(1–2):69–79.
59. Baixauli J, Delaney CP, Wu JS, et al. Functional outcome and quality of life after repeat ileal pouch-anal anastomosis for complications of ileoanal surgery. Dis Colon Rectum. 2004;47(1):2–11.
60. Dehni N, Remacle G, Dozois RR, et al. Salvage reoperation for complications after ileal pouch-anal anastomosis. Br J Surg. 2005;92(6):748–53.
61. Ortega-Deballon P, Cheynel N, Di-Giacomo G, et al. Interposition of a gastric pouch between ileum and anus after proctocolectomy: long-term results in 3 patients. Surgery. 2009;145(5):568–72.
62. Saltzberg SS, DiEdwardo C, Scott TE, et al. Ileal pouch salvage following failed ileal pouch-anal anastomosis. J Gastrointest Surg. 1999;3(6):633–41.

# Chapter 8
# Crohn's Disease in the Ileal Pouch Anal Anastomosis: Management Strategies

**Jonathan Segal and Ailsa Hart**

**Abstract** In patients with Crohn's disease,restorative proctocolectomy with ileo-anal anastomosis has been viewed as a relative contraindication. In selected patients, with appropriate counselling this approach may be considered. In some situations, Crohn's disease may be diagnosed months to years after formation of the pouch. This chapter aims to explore management strategies in patients with Crohn's disease and an ileoanal pouch as well as those with Crohn's disease considering an ileoanal pouch.

**Keywords** Crohn's disease · Fistulating disease · Pouch failure · Complication management · Quality of life · Treatment algorithm

## 8.1 Introduction

Since its introduction in 1978 the ileal pouch anal anastomosis is the surgery of choice for patients with ulcerative colitis (UC) refractory to medical therapy [1]. Restorative proctocolectomy (RPC) has been considered to be inappropriate in patients with an original diagnosis of Crohn's disease (CD) [2]. Reasons for this include an increased rate of pouch dysfunction, fistula formation, strictures of the pouch, abscess formation, peri-pouch sepsis and development of short bowel [3–5]. CD of the pouch is a poorly defined entity, and can be difficult to diagnose and challenging to treat [6].

Despite a high incidence of complications, several studies have demonstrated benefits of RPC for CD. Panis et al. [7] highlighted that in the absence of perianal or small bowel disease, RPC could be performed in patients with similar outcomes found in those who have a pouch for UC [7]. Regimbeau et al. [8] reported that in

J. Segal · A. Hart (✉)
St. Mark's Hospital, Harrow, UK

Imperial Healthcare NHS Trust, London, UK

Department of Surgery and Cancer, Imperial College, London, UK
e-mail: ailsa.hart@nhs.net

 
J. Warusavitarne, Z. Perry-Woodford (eds.), *The Ileoanal Pouch*,
https://doi.org/10.1007/978-3-319-94385-5_8

the absence of small bowel disease, RPC can be safely performed with limited morbidity at 10 year follow-up [8]. Phillips [2] suggests that it is unjustified to compare complication rates in RPC for CD with RPC for UC or FAP as they are completely different conditions. Phillips [2] highlights that any surgery for CD has more complications due to the nature of the disease and that RPC should not immediately be discounted in patients without small bowel or anal disease [2].

In view of this, the general approach to patients with known CD is to avoid RPC. In those who originally undergo RPC for presumed UC, the incidence of a change to a diagnosis of CD is 2–8% [5]. In patients with indeterminate colitis (IC), RPC is generally not considered due to concern that the disease will eventually develop into CD. Indeed, studies report that an initial diagnosis IC has a 15–20% of being changed to a diagnosis of CD after RPC [9].

Despite diagnostic advances, CD of the pouch can be difficult to detect and predict. In patients with RPC, *de novo* CD can develop weeks to years later, even when histopathological reassessment of the proctocolectomy clearly shows UC [10].

## 8.2 Defining CD of the Pouch

Patients with CD of the pouch can have a varied presentation. Symptoms often include abdominal pain, urgency, increased stool frequency, incontinence, seepage and extra-intestinal manifestations such as joint pains and rashes.

Criteria that have been used to diagnose CD of the pouch include: inflammation of the pouch that is resistant to antibiotic treatment, stricturing of the afferent limb, stricturing of the small bowel or fistulating disease [11–14].

Endoscopic assessment can help in the diagnosis of CD on pouchoscopy, but there is overlap in mucosal changes between CD of the pouch and pouchitis developing in UC. Features include discrete small and large mucosal ulcers, loss of vascular pattern, spontaneous bleeding and friability, exudates and inflammatory pseudopolyps in the pouch, cuff, or neo-terminal ileum [10]. The presence of pre-pouch ileitis (PPI) is controversial with some studies suggesting this may be an endoscopic feature of CD [15, 16]. PPI has no standard definition but is considered when there is inflammation that is proximal to the pouch. It has been reported that PPI occurs in patients with CD and not UC [15, 16]. In these studies, CD was defined as ulcerated lesions of the small bowel or afferent limb [15], or the presence of non-necrotising granulomas or transmural lymphoid aggregates in the colectomy specimen [16]. Other reports have suggested that PPI is not associated with CD [17].

Histological findings that help distinguish CD have been described. Weber et al. [18] found that pyloric gland metaplasia which was first described by Liber et al. [19] is a potential histological marker that can distinguish between chronic UC pouchitis and CD. Argarwal et al. [20] supported this finding and in addition suggested that high titres of anti-*Saccharomyces cerevisiae* antibody (ASCA) were associated with CD [20]. The presence of granulomas still represents the most accurate histological finding to help diagnose CD. Shen et al. [14] found that in only 10–20% of histological samples granulomas were found [14].

In conjunction with endoscopic and histological features, radiology can be a useful adjunct to help diagnose CD. The most common modalities used are MRI and CT scanning. These can help pick up small bowel strictures, the presence of fistulae and perianal disease which all may suggest a diagnosis of CD.

Despite advancing techniques such as metabomonic profiling, to date, there have been no biomarkers that have been found that help differentiate CD from other conditions in the pouch.

## 8.3 Aetiology of CD of the Pouch

In practice, CD of the pouch is often a post-operative diagnosis that develops in those patients who originally underwent restorative proctocolectomy for presumed ulcerative colitis. On the other hand, some patients with known CD pre-operatively never develop CD related complications of the pouch [21]. It remains unclear as to why some patients develop CD related complications of the pouch, however some authors have implicated the role of the microbiota in addition to surgery in creating an ideal "CD-friendly" environment [10]. Supporting this theory is the observation that many CD-like problems occur at the anastomosis and bowel segments proximal to the anastomosis [10]. This is the area in which the microbiota and local environment will undergo the most change [22].

Pre-operative risk factors for development of CD in the pouch have been highlighted. Melmed et al. [23] found that a positive family history of CD and the development of anti-Saccharomyces cerevisiae immunoglobulin-A seropositivity were significantly associated with a higher risk of developing CD complications following RPC [23]. Smoking has also been reported as a risk factor for developing CD of the pouch [24].

On a genetic level, it has been shown that polymorphisms for CD-like complications were in the 10q21 locus and the gene for PTGER4 [25]. A pre-operative diagnosis of IC [15, 26], younger age and female sex has been associated with fistulating CD [15].

Shen et al. [27] found significant association between the length of time a patient has a pouch and development of CD.

## 8.4 Classification of CD Complications

In order to manage CD-like complications, it is important that these patients are classified phenotypically to standardise investigations and management. CD-like complications can be grouped into inflammatory, stricturing, penetrating and perianal involvement. This is modified from the Vienna and Montreal classification of CD [28].

## 8.5 Differential Diagnosis

It is challenging to determine if pouch complications relate to an underlying diagnosis of CD, as often histological, radiological and symptoms can all overlap. Inflammation within the pouch can be caused by idiopathic pouchitis or secondary pouchitis driven by infection, ischaemia, medications, radiation, collagen deposition and NSAIDS [29]. The ability to determine the underlying diagnosis can be made more difficult due to idiopathic surgery-associated complications such as fistulae and sinuses that mimic clinical, endoscopic, and radiographic presentations of CD of the pouch [30].

### *8.5.1 Inflammation within the Pouch/ Pre-pouch Ileum*

Li et al. [30] suggested that features making a diagnosis of CD more likely are:

- The presence of a long segment of discrete/segmental involvement with inflammation (>10 cm) of the afferent limb which is often associated with concurrent pouch inlet or distal small bowel ulcerated strictures, in the absence of NSAID use.
- A difference in mucosal inflammation patterns between the pouch body and afferent limb can help distinguish CD from pouchitis with backwash ileitis in patients with PSC.
- The presence of ileitis or pouchitis that fails to respond to antibiotic therapy.
- Cuffitis refractory to topical therapy with mesalamine or corticosteroids.
- The presence of perianal lesions and perianal fistulae.
- Upper GI involvement.
- Active smoker.
- A family history of CD in one or more first-degree relatives.

### *8.5.2 Stricturing Disease*

Pouch strictures have an incidence as high as 12% [31], with a prevalence of pouch outlet strictures of 38% [32]. A greater number of strictures are observed after hand-sewn rather than stapled anastomoses [31]. The two common locations prone to strictures are the pouch outlet (i.e. at the pouch-anal anastomosis) [32] and the pouch inlet (i.e. at the junction of neo-terminal ileum and pouch). The most common causes of strictures besides CD of the pouch are anastomotic stenosis from surgery, ischaemia, and NSAID use [10] In practice, pouch outlet strictures are likely to be associated with surgical complications and ischaemia whereas pouch inlet strictures are likely to represent an inflammatory process and therefore are more likely to be associated with CD.

### *8.5.3 Small Bowel Obstruction*

The incidence of small bowel obstruction following RPC ranges from 13% to 35% [33–36]. Causes of small bowel obstruction in pouches include adhesions following surgery, sepsis and CD of the small bowel.

### *8.5.4 Fistulating Disease*

Fistulating disease of the pouch carries significant morbidity and is a major cause of pouch failure [37]. The presence of fistulating disease does not necessarily confirm a diagnosis of CD as surgical complications such as wound dehiscence, anastomotic leaks and iatrogenic bowel injury can contribute to fistulating disease.

Pouch fistulae may occur at any time following restorative proctocolectomy, with an incidence of 2.6–14%, depending on the length of follow-up [38–41]. Fistulae have been associated with a high chance of pouch failure, with studies suggesting a pouch failure rate of 21–30% following fistula formation in the pouch [40–42]. Common locations of fistulae include pouch-vaginal fistulae, perianal fistulae, pouch-cutaneous fistulae and pouch-bladder fistulae [30].

The timing of fistula formation can help aid in the diagnosis, with early fistula formation in a patient with presumed UC, more likely to represent a complication following surgery with later fistula formation in the absence of sepsis and leaks more likely to represent an inflammatory process such as CD [43, 44].

Anatomical location can also help determine the aetiology of the pouch fistula. Pouch fistulae associated with the anastomosis are more likely to represent surgical aetiology whereas more complex fistulae including those found in the anal canal are likely to be more associated with CD [10].

Furthermore, response to medical treatments including antibiotics and biologics has been suggested to be an important factor in aiding diagnosis [6]. Fistulae that respond to these medical therapies are likely to be inflammatory in nature [6].

### *8.5.5 Pouch-Vaginal Fistulae*

The overall risk of pouch-vaginal fistulae after RPC varies between 4% and 16%, with pouch failure occurring in 21–30% of these patients [45]. The natural history of pouch vaginal fistulae has been poorly studied; however it has been reported that these are strongly associated with CD of the pouch [46–48]. Heriot et al. [49] found that the majority of pouch vaginal fistulae (76%) originated from the pouch-anal anastomosis. Surgical risk factors include injury to the vagina or rectovaginal septum during pelvic dissection [50], J-pouch design [51], hand sewn anastomosis [44], entrapment from the circular stapling device [52], anastomotic dehiscence and pelvic sepsis [47].

## 8.6 Management of CD of the Pouch

The literature on the management of CD of the pouch is scant, with most of the evidence from small case series. General preventative advice includes avoidance of cigarette smoking and NSAID use [53]. Studies have yet to determine the long-term impact biologics have on pouch survival.

### 8.6.1 *Inflammation*

The underlying aetiology driving pouch inflammation can be difficult to ascertain. Many patients with inflammation within the pouch will be treated empirically with a course of antibiotics in the first instance for presumed idiopathic pouchitis [54]. If antibiotic treatment fails, other diagnoses are considered with the aid of investigations.

Limited literature suggests that CD and cuffitis of the pouch can be treated with topical 5-aminosalicylate agents, oral or topical corticosteroids, antibiotics, and immunomodulators [10]. Biologics have been considered treatment for CD in the pouch, with a study showing that biologics can be effective in 84–88% [55–57]. The conclusions we can draw from these studies are limited as sub-group analysis reporting treatment outcomes for confirmed CD of the pouch was not reported. In these studies, the patient populations were heterogeneous with efficacy of treatment reported in patients with fistulating CD, medically refractory pouchitis and pouchitis associated with ulcerative colitis.

### 8.6.2 *Strictures*

Management of pouch strictures includes medication, endoscopic balloon dilation [58], bougie dilatation under general anaesthetic [32] and in the case of pouch outlet strictures, self-dilatation at home [31]. If pouch strictures are severe, the stricture may result in bowel obstruction, evacuation problems, pouch dilatation, and bacterial overgrowth [59]. Furthermore, it has been reported that pouch strictures were commonly associated with intraoperative or postoperative complications, which often necessitated surgical therapy to salvage pouch function, and are eventually responsible for pouch failure [31].

Endoscopic balloon dilatation has been extensively used for the treatment of fibrostenotic CD [60] with limited data on its efficacy and safety for use in pouch-related strictures related to CD of the pouch [58]. Shen et al. [61] found that balloon dilatation for pouch strictures was effective, safe and associated with a 5- 10-, and 25-year pouch retention/survival rates of 97%, 90.6%, and 85.9%, respectively. Within this cohort they found that an underlying diagnosis of CD was associated with an increased chance of pouch failure (Hazard ratio 1.61 (0.99–2.61) $p = 0.05$) [61].

Surgical treatment options include pouch excision, stricturoplasty, reconstruction, or a proximal diverting stoma [31, 32, 62]. All but stricturoplasty can be considered as pouch failure. Wu et al. [63] is the only study comparing both stricturoplasty with balloon dilatation and found survival rates of 83.1 and 82.0% for patients with stricturoplasty and endoscopic dilation, respectively (log-rank test: $p = 0.752$). They also found that CD on univariate analysis was associated with a stricture free survival ($p = 0.02$). This study recommended the use of balloon dilatation in the first instance for pouch strictures with surgical stricturoplasty reserved for refractory cases. All other management strategies have not been compared for efficacy and safety.

### *8.6.3 Small Bowel Obstruction*

The management of small bowel obstruction in a CD pouch has been poorly studied but these should be managed in a similar fashion to any small bowel obstruction. MacLean et al. [34] suggested that these rarely require any operative form of treatment and can be managed conservatively [34].

We suggest that patients with suspected small bowel obstruction need urgent investigations. Whilst awaiting investigations early surgical opinion is important. Early investigations include bloods, abdominal and erect chest x-rays to rule out perforation. Early cross sectional imaging will also be vital to help the diagnosis.

Initial treatment may include making the patient nil by mouth, intravenous fluids and decompression of the stomach with a nasogastric tube. In CD of the pouch, an underlying inflammatory process may be the underlying cause of intestinal obstruction. In this situation, a trial of medical therapy to include steroids, antibiotics or biologics may help reduce inflammation and resolve the obstruction. Endoscopic therapy can include endoscopic dilatation and stenting. Surgical techniques such as stricturoplasties and bowel resection can also be considered.

### *8.6.4 Fistulae*

The treatment of fistulae in CD of the pouch is based on small case series. Ricart et al. [64] reported that four of the five patients (80%) with fistulae had a complete response with sustained closure of all fistulae with infliximab [64].This was further supported by Viazis [65] who reported a 66.7% complete fistulae closure in patients given 1 year of infliximab. Gaertner et al. [66] whilst they could not compare efficacy of each management strategy, found that seton insertion and lay-open fistulotomy were associated with high healing rates in fistulae [66].

### 8.6.5 Pouch Vaginal Fistulae

Pouch vaginal fistulae can be managed using medical and surgical approaches. Ricart et al. [64] found that infliximab caused complete remission in a third of patients who had pouch vaginal fistulae [64]. A case series by Koroos [67] highlighted that CD paediatric pouch vaginal fistulae could be healed with infliximab. Surgical options include primary repair of the transvaginal fistula with healing rates reported as 55% when done as a primary procedure and 40% when performed secondarily [68]. Shah et al. [50] supported local repair following pouch vaginal fistulae, they achieved pouch vaginal fistula closure using local repairs in addition to medical therapy, setons, and stomas [50] with an overall healing rate of 52% at 49-month mean follow-up. Heriot et al. [49] supported these findings, reporting outcomes in 37 patients (54%) who underwent local transvaginal repair, they found primary healing rate was 40% at a median follow-up of 19 months, with an overall pouch failure rate of 35% at a median of 4.2 years [49].

Mallick et al. [68] reported that local repair with pouch advancement flap was associated with a healing rate of 55% when done as a primary procedure and 40% when performed secondarily after a different procedure, which included ileal pouch advancement flap and transvaginal approach to repair [68]. They highlighted that pouch failure was higher in patients with CD who underwent primary surgical repair compared with non-CD patients with pouch vaginal fistulae. Despite seemingly good results, the authors strongly recommended faecal diversion in the management of pouch vaginal fistula as the authors felt that this gave the best chance of resolution of sepsis and inflammation [68]. In this study, a delayed diagnosis of CD was made in 24 patients, and these patients had lower success rates following ileal advancement flaps compared with the non-Crohn's group (25 vs. 48%). Other studies have used EUA, setons and glue successfully in pouch vaginal fistulae [69].

Based on their experience, Gaertner et al. [66] proposed the following treatment algorithm for management of ileal pouch fistulae [66] (Fig. 8.1).

### 8.6.6 Pouch Failure

Despite attempts to salvage a CD pouch, it has been estimated that pouch excision rates are 45–55% in patients with pre-operative CD [5, 9]. Whilst there is no absolute indication for pouch excision in CD of the pouch, we suggest that a joint decision with the patient and the multi-disciplinary team to include physicians, surgeons and nurses are essential. Reasons to consider pouch failure include; symptoms which are not tolerable to the patient, medically refractory disease, signs of persistent metabolic disease, failure to thrive, malnourishment, and overall poor quality of life. In this instance, pouch excision or an ileostomy should be offered.

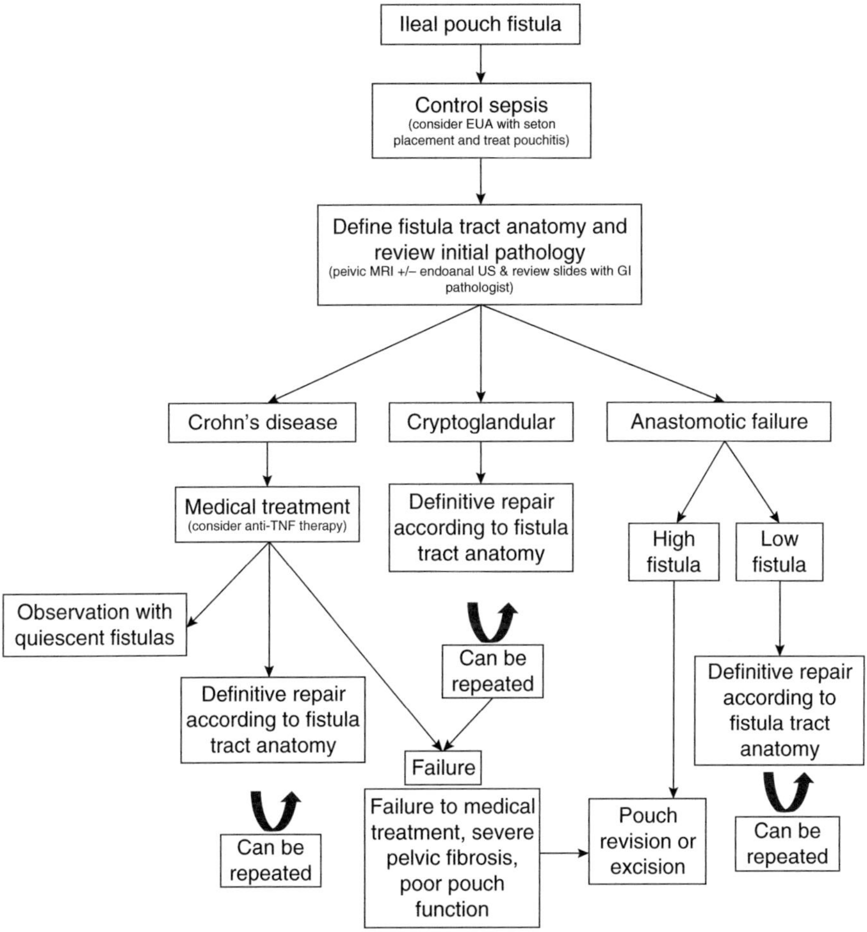


**Fig. 8.1** Treatment algorithm for management of ileal pouch fistulae (Gaertner et al. [66])

## 8.7 Prognosis of CD of the Pouch

In a cohort of 32 patients with CD of the pouch, 93% of patients developed complications including abscesses, pouchitis, and strictures and 29% of these patients had pouch failure [70] secondary to these complications. Of those patients who retained their pouch 60% had leakage, with 45% using pads. Gu et al. [71] reported a 5 and 10 year pouch retention rate of 58% and 50%, respectively [71]. This included 17 patients who had inflammatory CD, 7 had who fibrostenotic disease, and 41 had fistulising phenotype.

In a small study comparing RPC for UC vs RPC for CD, the CD group experienced significantly fewer median daily bowel movements (p = 0.02), with less episodes of incontinence for liquids ($p < 0.01$) and less episodes of pouchitis ($p < 0.01$). However, pouch excision rates are significantly higher in the CD group (2 vs 0%, $p < 0.01$) [72].

Overall, understanding CD in restorative proctocolectomy in terms of its benefits, risks and treatment options remains very limited. A consensus definition of CD of the pouch will be beneficial to future study designs in addition to being able to understand and separate CD complications of the pouch from other non-CD complications. This will allow future trials to specifically address CD complications and assess treatment affect for that specific complication. Further randomized control trials are likely to require multi-centre approach due to relatively small numbers.

## References

1. Parks AG, Nicholls RJ. Proctocolectomy without ileostomy for ulcerative colitis. Br Med J. 1978;2:85–8.
2. Phillips RK. Ileal pouch-anal anastomosis for Crohn's disease. Gut. 1998;43:303–4.
3. Hartley JE, et al. Analysis of the outcome of ileal pouch-anal anastomosis in patients with Crohn's disease. Dis Colon Rectum. 2004;47:1808–15.
4. Brown CJ, et al. Crohn's disease and indeterminate colitis and the ileal pouch-anal anastomosis: outcomes and patterns of failure. Dis Colon Rectum. 2005;48:1542–9.
5. Yu CS, Pemberton JH, Larson D. Ileal pouch-anal anastomosis in patients with indeterminate colitis: long-term results. Dis Colon Rectum. 2000;43:1487–96.
6. Lightner AL, Pemberton JH, Loftus EJ. Crohn's disease of the ileoanal pouch. Inflamm Bowel Dis. 2016;22:1502–8.
7. Panis Y, et al. Ileal pouch/anal anastomosis for Crohn's disease. Lancet. 1996;347:854–7.
8. Regimbeau JM, et al. Long-term results of ileal pouch-anal anastomosis for colorectal Crohn's disease. Dis Colon Rectum. 2001;44:769–78.
9. Keighley MR. The final diagnosis in pouch patients for presumed ulcerative colitis may change to Crohn's disease: patients should be warned of the consequences. Acta Chir Iugosl. 2000;47:27–31.
10. Shen B. Crohn's disease of the ileal pouch: reality, diagnosis, and management. Inflamm Bowel Dis. 2009;15:284–94.
11. Deutsch AA, McLeod RS, Cullen J, Cohen Z. Results of the pelvic-pouch procedure in patients with Crohn's disease. Dis Colon Rectum. 1991;34:475–7.
12. Grobler SP, Hosie KB, Keighley MRB. Randomized trial of loop ileostomy in restorative proctocolectomy. Br J Surg. 1992;79:903–6.
13. Hyman NH, Fazio VW, Tuckson WB, Lavery IC. Consequences of ileal pouch-anal anastomosis for Crohn's colitis. Dis Colon Rectum. 1991;34:653–7.
14. Shen B, et al. Clinical features and quality of life in patients with different phenotypes of Crohn's disease of the ileal pouch. Dis Colon Rectum. 2007;50:1450–9.
15. Shen B, et al. Risk factors for clinical phenotypes of Crohn's disease of the ileal pouch. Am J Gastroenterol. 2006;101:2760–8.
16. Wolf JM, et al. Afferent limb ulcers predict Crohn's disease in patients with ileal pouch-anal anastomosis. Gastroenterology. 2004;126:1686–91.
17. McLaughlin SD, et al. Incidence and short-term implications of prepouch ileitis following restorative proctocolectomy with ileal pouch-anal anastomosis for ulcerative colitis. Dis Colon Rectum. 2009;52:879–83.
18. Weber CR, Rubin DT. Chronic pouchitis versus recurrent Crohn's disease: a diagnostic challenge. Dig Dis Sci. 2013;58:2748–50.
19. Liber AF. Aberrant pyloric glands in regional ileitis. AMA Arch Pathol. 1951;51:205–12 (

20. Agarwal S, et al. Is pyloric gland metaplasia in ileal pouch biopsies a marker for Crohn's disease? Dig Dis Sci. 2013;58:2918–25.
21. Shen B, Patel S, Lian I. Natural history of Crohn's disease in patients who underwent intentional restorative proctocolectomy with ileal pouch-anal anastomosis. Aliment Pharmacol Ther. 2009;31:745–53.
22. Guyton K, Alverdy JC. The gut microbiota and gastrointestinal surgery. Nat Rev Gastroenterol Hepatol. 2016;14:43–54.
23. Melmed GY, et al. Family history and serology predict Crohn's disease after ileal pouch-anal anastomosis for ulcerative colitis. Dis Colon Rectum. 2008;51:100–8.
24. Shen B, et al. Risk factors for diseases of ileal pouch-anal anastomosis after restorative proctocolectomy for ulcerative colitis. Clin Gastroenterol Hepatol. 2006;4:81-9–3.
25. Sehgal R, et al. Genetic risk profiling and gene signature modeling to predict risk of complications after IPAA. Dis Colon Rectum. 2012;55:239–48.
26. Delaney CP, Remzi FH, Gramlich T, Dadvand B, Fazio VW. Equivalent function, quality of life and pouch survival rates after ileal pouch-anal anastomosis for indeterminate and ulcerative colitis. Ann Surg. 2002;236:43–8.
27. Shen B, et al. Risk factors for diseases of ileal pouch–anal anastomosis after restorative proctocolectomy for ulcerative colitis. Clin Gastroenterol Hepatol. 2006;4:81–9.
28. Satsangi J, Silverberg MS, Vermeire S, Colombel J-F. The Montreal classification of inflammatory bowel disease: controversies, consensus, and implications. Gut. 2006;55: 749–53.
29. Navaneethan U, Shen B. U., N. Secondary pouchitis: those with identifiable etiopathogenetic or triggering factors. Am J Gastroenterol. 2010;105:51–64.
30. Li Y, Wu B, Shen B. Diagnosis and differential diagnosis of Crohn's disease of the ileal pouch. Curr Gastroenterol Rep. 2012;14:406–13.
31. Prudhomme M, Dozois RR, Godlewski G, Mathison S, Fabbro-Peray P. Anal canal strictures after ileal pouch-anal anastomosis. Dis Colon Rectum. 1996;676:20–3.
32. Lewis WG, Kuzu A, Sagar PM, Holdsworth PJ, Johnston D. Stricture at the pouch-anal anastomosis after restorative proctocolectomy. Dis Colon Rectum. 1994;37(2):120–5.
33. Fazio VW, et al. Ileal pouch-anal anastomoses complications and function in 1005 patients. Ann Surg. 1995;222:120–7.
34. MacLean AR, et al. Risk of small bowel obstruction after the ileal pouch-anal anastomosis. Ann Surg. 2002;235:200–6.
35. Young CJ, et al. Evolution of the pelvic pouch procedure at one institution: the first 100 cases. Aust N Z J Surg. 1999;69:438–42.
36. Marcello PW, et al. Obstruction after ileal pouch-anal anastomosis: a preventable complication? Dis Colon Rectum. 1993;36:1105–11.
37. Haveran LA, et al. Infliximab and/or azathioprine in the treatment of Crohn's disease-like complications after IPAA. Dis Colon Rectum. 2011;54:15–20.
38. Hahnloser D, et al. Results at up to 20 years after ileal pouch-anal anastomosis for chronic ulcerative colitis. Br J Surg. 2007;94:333–40.
39. Breen EM, et al. Functional results after perineal complications of ileal pouch-anal anastomosis. Dis Colon Rectum. 1998;41:691–5.
40. Fazio VW, et al. Quantification of risk for pouch failure after ileal pouch anal anastomosis surgery. Ann Surg. 2003;238:605–14–7.
41. Tekkis PP, et al. Risk factors associated with ileal pouch-related fistula following restorative proctocolectomy. Br J Surg. 2005;92:1270–6.
42. Nisar PJ, Kiran RP, Shen B, Remzi FH, Fazio VW. Factors associated with Ileoanal pouch failure in patients developing early or late pouch-related fistula. Dis Colon Rectum. 2011;54:446–53.
43. Tekkis PP, et al. Long-term outcomes of restorative proctocolectomy for Crohn's disease and indeterminate colitis. Colorectal Dis. 2005;7:218–23.
44. Lee PY, et al. Vaginal fistula following restorative proctocolectomy. Dis Colon Rectum. 1997;40:752–9.

45. Lolohea S, Lynch AC, Robertson GB, Frizelle FA. Ileal pouch-anal anastomosis-vaginal fistula: a review. Dis Colon Rectum. 2005;48:1802–10.
46. Wexner SD, et al. Ileal pouch vaginal fistulae: incidence, etiology, and management. Dis Colon Rectum. 1989;32:460–5.
47. Keighley MR, Grobler SP. Fistula complicating restorative proctocolectomy. Br J Surg. 1993;80:1065–7.
48. Melton GB, et al. Long-term outcomes with ileal pouch-anal anastomosis and Crohn's disease. Trans Meet Am Surg Assoc. 2008;126:251–9.
49. Heriot AG, et al. Management and outcome of pouch-vaginal fistulae following restorative proctocolectomy. Dis Colon Rectum. 2005;48:451–8.
50. Shah NS, Remzi F, Massmann A, Baixauli J, Fazio VW. Management and treatment outcome of pouch-vaginal fistulae following restorative proctocolectomy. Dis Colon Rectum. 2003;46:911–7.
51. Groom JS, Nicholls RJ, Hawley PR, Phillips RK. Pouch-vaginal fistula. Br J Surg. 1993;80:936–40.
52. Sagar PM, Pemberton JH. Intraoperative, postoperative and reoperative problems with ileoanal pouches. Br J Surg. 2012;99:454–68.
53. Shen B. Diagnosis and management of postoperative ileal pouch disorders. Clin Colon Rectal Surg. 2010;23:259–68.
54. Segal JP, et al. Systematic review with meta-analysis: the management of chronic refractory pouchitis with an evidence-based treatment algorithm. Aliment Pharmacol Ther. 2016. https://doi.org/10.1111/apt.13905.
55. Barreiro-de Acosta M, et al. Efficacy of infliximab rescue therapy in patients with chronic refractory pouchitis: a multicenter study. Inflamm Bowel Dis. 2012;18:812–7.
56. Colombel J-F, et al. Management of Crohn's disease of the ileoanal pouch with infliximab. Am J Gastroenterol. 2003;98:2239–44.
57. Ferrante M, et al. Efficacy of infliximab in refractory pouchitis and Crohn's disease-related complications of the pouch: a belgian case series. Inflamm Bowel Dis. 2010;16:243–9.
58. Shen B, et al. Endoscopic balloon dilation of ileal pouch strictures. Am J Gastroenterol. 2004;99:2340–7.
59. Gorgun E, Remzi FH. Complications of ileoanal pouches. Clin Colon Rectal Surg. 2004;17:43–55.
60. Navaneethan U, Lourdusamy V, Njei B, Shen B. Endoscopic balloon dilation in the management of strictures in Crohn's disease: a systematic review and meta-analysis of non-randomized trials. Surg Endosc. 2016; https://doi.org/10.1007/s00464-016-4902-1.
61. Shen B, et al. Efficacy and safety of endoscopic treatment of ileal pouch strictures. Inflamm Bowel Dis. 2011;17:2527–35.
62. MacLean AR, O'Connor B, Parkes R, Cohen Z, McLeod RS. Reconstructive surgery for failed ileal pouch-anal anastomosis: a viable surgical option with acceptable results. Dis Colon Rectum. 2002;45:880–6.
63. Wu X, Mukewar S, Kiran RP, Remzi FH, Shen B. Surgical stricturoplasty in the treatment of ileal pouch strictures. J Gastrointest Surg. 2013;17:1452–61.
64. Ricart E, et al. Successful management of Crohn's disease of the ileoanal pouch with infliximab. Gastroenterology. 1999;117:429–32.
65. Viazis N, et al. One-year infliximab administration for the treatment of chronic refractory pouchitis. Ann Gastroenterol. 2011;24:290–3.
66. Gaertner WB, et al. Ileal pouch fistulae after restorative proctocolectomy: management and outcomes. Tech Coloproctol. 2014;18:1061–6.
67. Kooros K, Katz AJ. Infliximab therapy in pediatric Crohn's pouchitis. Inflamm Bowel Dis. 2004;10:417–20.
68. Mallick IH, Hull TL, Remzi FH, Kiran RP. Management and outcome of pouch-vaginal fistulae after IPAA surgery. Dis Colon Rectum. 2014;57:490–6.

69. Tsujinaka S, et al. Surgical management of pouch-vaginal fistula after restorative proctocolectomy. J Am Coll Surg. 2006;202:912–8.
70. Braveman JM, et al. The fate of the ileal pouch in patients developing Crohn's disease. Dis Colon Rectum. 2004;47:1613–9.
71. Gu J, Stocchi L, Kiran RP, Shen B, Remzi FH. Do clinical characteristics of de novo pouch Crohn's disease after restorative proctocolectomy affect ileal pouch retention? Dis Colon Rectum. 2014;57:76–82.
72. Grucela AL, Bauer JJ, Gorfine SR, Chessin DB. Outcome and long-term function of restorative proctocolectomy for Crohn's disease: comparison to patients with ulcerative colitis. Colorectal Dis. 2011;13:426–30.

# Chapter 9
# Microbiology of the Ileoanal Pouch and Managing Pouchitis

**Simon McLaughlin**

**Abstract** Pouchitis is the most common cause of pouch dysfunction occurring in 20–50% of patients following restorative proctocolectomy for ulcerative colits (UC). In 6% of patients the inflammation extends proximal to the pouch; pre-pouch ileitis. The inflammation that occurs in patients with pouchitis is likely secondary to the combination of a dysregulated immune system that exists in all patients with UC and a stimulus from the gut microbiota.

The mainstay of treatment is antibiotic therapy which is likely to be effective by reducing total gut microbial load and therefore stimulus to the immune system. In those who do not respond or lose response to this treatment there is evidence for the development of antibiotic resistant bacteria and changing antibiotic class is often effective. In those refractory to antibiotics biologic therapy can be effective.

**Keywords** Pouchitis · Pre-pouch ileitis · Restorative proctocoelctomy · Biologics Probiotics

## 9.1 Introduction

Restorative proctolectomy (RPC) with ileal-pouch anal anastomosis is the operation of choice for patients who require surgery for ulcerative colitis (UC). Following surgery expected bowel frequency is 4–8 times per day and 0–2 overnight. This frequency increases in patients with pouch dysfunction. Pouchitis is the most common cause of pouch dysfunction occurring in 20–50% of patients [1–3]. It usually presents with an increase in stool frequency and urgency, some patients will also develop abdominal cramping, fever and per-anal bleeding. To correctly diagnose

S. McLaughlin
The Royal Bournemouth and Christchurch Hospitals NHS foundation trust, Bournemouth, UK

Centre of Postgraduate Research and Medical Education, Bournemouth University, Poole, UK
e-mail: simon.mclaughlin@nhs.net

 
J. Warusavitarne, Z. Perry-Woodford (eds.), *The Ileoanal Pouch*,
https://doi.org/10.1007/978-3-319-94385-5_9

pouchitis and exclude other conditions baseline tests should include stool tests to exclude common pathogens including C. difficile.

A flexible pouchoscopy with intubation of the pre-pouch ileum is essential. In some patients the inflammation will be found to extend proximal to the pouch; pre-pouch ileitis.

## 9.2 Microbiological Aetiology

Whether a dysbiosis (altered gut microbiota composition) or an abnormal host immune response to normal commensal microbiota is the cause of inflammatory bowel disease has been the subject of a large number of studies. Considerable evidence from clinical practice implicate bacteria in the pathogenesis of pouchitis; pouchitis occurs in the area of the small bowel with the highest concentration of bacteria, antibiotics are effective treatment for treating pouchitis and probiotics can prevent the onset of pouchitis and reduce disease relapse.

The hypothesis that an abnormal immune response is fundamental to the disease process that occurs in all forms of IBD is well established [4]. In pouchitis this is demonstrated by the knowledge that the incidence of pouchitis in familial adenomatous polyposis (FAP) patients is about 10 times less common than in patients with a history of ulcerative colitis suggesting that the increased risk in UC patients may be due to an abnormal immune system.

Around 99% of gut microbiota are contained in four phyla; Firmicutes, Bacteroidetes, Proteobacteria and Actinobacteria [5, 6]. At the species level however, each individual has his or her own unique gut microbiota, It has been appreciated for about 10 years that 90% of gut microbiota cannot be cultured [5] and therefore molecular biology techniques (16s ribosomal RNA polymerase chain reaction) are required to accurately identify the composition of gut microbiota. Data from early culture-based techniques must therefore be disregarded and will not be discussed here.

Following closure of ileostomy the pouch microbiota evolve over at least the first year and differ between patients. In a study by Falk et al. two patients underwent repeated pouch mucosal biopsy [7]. The microbiota were identified using terminal restriction fragment length polymorphism (T-RFLP), cloning and sequencing, the microbiotal composition evolved over time and at 1 year was broadly similar to that found in the normal colon.

A reduction in bacterial diversity is thought to be fundamental to the pathogenesis of all forms of IBD. Kubacher et al. identified a reduction in diversity in patients with a history of chronic pouchitis who had a relapse of pouchitis following an antibiotic induced remission when compared to patients maintained on the probiotic VSL#3 who remained in remission [8].

In the probiotic treated patients increases in the diversity of Lactobacilli and Bifidobacteria were identified.

It is recognised that gastroenteritis secondary to pathogenic bacteria such as campylobacter and C.difficile can mimic a new presentation of IBD and also cause a flare of symptoms in patients with known IBD. CMV infection is unusual in patients not immunosuppressed but silent carriage is not uncommon. One group identified CMV in biopsies taken from both pouchitis and non-pouchitis pouch patients using a polymerase chain reaction (PCR) and sequencing technique. No significant difference was found in the incidence of CMV in each group when classified using the modified pouch disease activity index suggesting that CMV is unlikely to be implicated in the pathogenesis of pouchitis [9].

Six studies have compared the differences in the microbiota in pouchitis and non-pouchitis RPC patients using molecular biology techniques with differing results.

The earliest study by Komanduri et al. paradoxically reported an increase in the bacterial diversity in pouch biopsy samples from pouchitis patients compared to biopsies from the ileum of non IBD controls with an intact colon. There was an increase in the proportion of proteobacteria and a reduction in firmicutes as well as a difference in the Rumicoccus species associated with pouchitis (R. obeum) and non-pouchitis (R. gnavus) [10].

These findings are at odds to other IBD studies and should be interpreted with caution as there were significant limitations to this study. Bacterial analysis was undertaken by grouping biopsy samples together by disease type rather than by analysing each patient sample individually. It therefore remains possible that the identified differences could have been from single patient samples within each group. Furthermore according to the authors' the technique at most identified 73% of the microbial population.

An early study from the St. Mark's group used a hybrid culture and molecular biology technique where mucosal biopsies were first cultured on agar before bacteria were extracted and amplified using PCR and profiles were generated using TRFLP [11]. No differences between pouchitis and non-pouchitis groups or FAP and UC groups were identified. It should however be appreciated that the culturing of biopsies before PCR would favour growth of bacteria supported by the culture medium and influence the results of PCR. In addition, the TRFLP technique can only identify dominant species groups and cannot identify individual bacterial species.

A further study by Lim et al. utilised the TRFLP technique to compare pouchitis (5 UC patients) and non-pouchitis (15 UC patients). No differences in diversity or TRFLP profile were identified between groups [12].

In 2008 the St. Mark's group reported the results of the first study that identified the microbiota in pouchitis and non pouchitis UC patients and compared this to pouchitis and non pouchitis FAP patients using a 16s rRNA sequencing technique [13]. In total 24 patients were studied (patients with antibiotic resistant pouchitis were excluded) the results identified a significant increase in Proteobacteria and a significant reduction in Bacteroidetes and *Faecalibacterium prausnitzii* in the total UC compared with the total FAP group. Similar findings have been reported in a study which compared the microbiota in IBD and non-IBD surgical specimens [5], suggesting that a similar dysbiosis exists in all types of IBD. This study also demonstrated that the ileal pouch microbiota differed from those expected in the normal colon; *Proteobacteria* usually account for a small proportion of colonic microbiota in non IBD patients but up to 20% in IBD patients [5] in this study proteobacteria accounted for a median of 66.6% of the microbiota in UC RPC patients. Lower proportions of *Bacteriodetes, Lachnospiraceae* and *Ruminococcaceae* were also identified. Other IBD studies have also identified increases in *Proteobacteria* suggesting that a similar dysbiosis is implicated in the pathogenesis of the inflammatory process that occurs in patients with UC before and after RPC. Further findings in this study were a reduction in bacterial diversity in UC patients (both with and without pouchitis) compared to FAP patients and a further reduction in diversity when UC pouchitis samples were compared to UC non-pouchitis samples. This observation complements Kulbacher et al.'s study) [8] (described earlier) that an increased bacterial diversity was found in those with a history of pouchitis who remained in remission with the probiotic VSL#3. Again a reduction in diversity has been identified in non-pouch IBD studies providing further evidence that this is a key predisposing factor to the development of IBD and treatments that aim to increase diversity may reverse or prevent gut inflammation.

Reshef et al. performed the largest study to date using 16s rRNA sequencing [14]. 140 patients (131 UC, 9 FAP) were recruited and followed up over 18 months, 38 with a normal pouch, 83 pouchitis (37 of which had chronic pouchitis) and 10 whose classification changed during follow-up. 120 samples were taken from patients prior to first treatment with antibiotics. The authors' analysed faecal samples (rather than biopsy specimens). Similar to the St. Mark's study the authors' identified a reduction in bacterial diversity in those with pouchitis when compared to non-pouchitis samples and only minor differences in microbiota composition including a reduction in *Faecalibacterium* in those with pouchitis.

A recent study from the Leuven group identified the microbiota in faecal samples before and after colectomy and compared pouchitis and non-pouchitis patients. The authors report that the presence of R. gnavus, B. vulgatus, C. perfringens and the absence of Blautia and Roseburia in faecal samples in patients before colectomy is associated with an increased risk of developing pouchitis [15]. This could fit well with the concept that probiotics reduce the risk of developing pouchitis in the first year following RPC [16].

## 9.3 Treatment of Pouchitis

Pouchitis usually presents with an increase in stool frequency and urgency. Some patients will also develop abdominal cramping, fever and per-anal bleeding. Before initiating treatment stool tests should be performed to exclude an enteric infection including C. difficile. Flexible pouchoscopy including intubation and biopsy of the pre-pouch ileum should be undertaken to confirm pouchitis. Features that should raise the suspicion of Crohn's disease (CD) include patchy pouch inflammation with intervening normal mucosa and inflammation of the pre-pouch ileum that is not contiguous ie. normal intervening mucosa with preserved vascular pattern. Pre-pouch ileitis occurs in about 6% of pouchitis patients [17] and has distinct histological characteristics [18].

It should be appreciated that in common with mainstream IBD pathognomic histological findings of CD from biopsies are uncommon even in patients where this is the final diagnosis. In these patients video capsule endoscopy may be helpful to document the true extent of small bowel inflammation and this may reduce diagnostic uncertainty in patients with suspected CD. Confirming the final histopathological diagnosis at colectomy is always important; the likelihood of missed CD being higher in those with genuine indeterminate colitis. In patients where there is difficulty differentiating between a diagnosis of pre-pouch ileitis and CD a therapeutic trial of combination antibiotic therapy is useful since the response rate in those with pre-pouch ileitis is high and this therapy is both safe and cheap.

## 9.4 Antibiotic Therapy

Antibiotic treatment with oral ciprofloxacin 500 mg twice daily or metronidazole 400 mg three times daily for 2 weeks is first line treatment. Topical metronidazole may be useful in those who fail ciprofloxacin and develop intolerable side effects to oral metronidazole. If refractory to a single antibiotic agent then ciprofloxacin combined with metronidazole/tinidazole/rifaximin is usually effective [19]. In those patients who do not respond to this treatment then faecal coliform sensitivity testing should be performed and antibiotic selection based on the results of the sensitivity patterns.

## 9.5 Oral Steroid and Sulphasalazine Treatment

Budesonide in two open label studies from the same centre has been reported to be effective with clinical remission reported in 15 of 20 (75%) patients treated with 9 mg oral budesonide once daily for 8 weeks and 8 of 10 (80%) in those treated with oral beclomethasone dipropionate 10 mg daily [20].

In an open label study of 11 patients suphasalzine 1 g three times daily was effective with 63% of patients in remission after 8 weeks of treatment and may be an alternative to antibiotics [21].

## 9.6 Immunosuppressants and Biologics

Seven studies have reported the efficacy of biologic drugs to treat refractory pouchitis. Clinical remission in those treated with infliximab varied between 27–100% and 13–72% in those treated with adalimumab [19].

Topical tacrolimus has been reported to be effective. In a single open label study 7 of 10 patients were in a clinical remission after 8 weeks of once daily therapy [22].

Alicaforsen an antisense inhibitor of ICAM-1 has been proposed as a novel treatment for IBD however to date published data in UC and CD patients with intact colons demonstrate low efficacy [23]. In pouchitis clinical improvement in 11 of 13 patients following treatment with 240 mg enemas for 6 weeks has been reported in one retrospective study of data from 3 referral centres in Switzerland. Unfortunately, remission was not sustained and 81.8% of patients relapsed after therapy was withdrawn. In two patients that were given a second treatment course a more prolonged remission was reported and the authors suggest that maintenance therapy or prolonged treatment may be required. Alicaforsen is not currently licensed in the UK.

Azathioprine appears ineffective with reports of patients with PSC receiving this drug following liver transplantation developing pouchitis [24, 25].

## 9.7 Novel Therapies

The evidence for other treatments is limited. Novel treatments including bismuth enema [26], elemental diet (E028) [27] and faecal microbial transplant appear to be ineffective [28].

## 9.8 Pre-pouch Ileitis

To date two studies have specifically assessed the outcome of treatment in patients with pre-pouch ileitis. In a study of 14 patients 86% were in a clinical remission after combination antibiotic therapy with 500 mg ciprofloxacin twice daily and metronidazole 400 mg twice daily for 4 weeks [29].

Infliximab has also been reported to be effective in seven patients with chronic pouchitis and pre-pouch ileitis, 86% of patients were in a clinical remission following 3 infliximab infusions [30]. The results of this study should be interpreted with caution as the authors' reported extensive small bowel inflammation identified at video capsule endoscopy which raises the possibility of CD although this was not confirmed at histology.

## 9.9 Maintenance Therapy

In those patients where remission has been achieved with biologic drugs then it is reasonable to continue this therapy in line with usual IBD clinical guidelines.

In those patients who respond to antibiotics but have three or more episodes of pouchitis per year or relapse on withdrawal of antibiotics maintenance therapy is recommended [31].

Maintenance treatment with antibiotics appears safe, effective and improves quality of life at least in the medium term. In a study of 25 patients receiving maintenance antibiotic therapy (median length of treatment of 15.8 months) at St. Mark's hospital the only complication reported was the development of vaginal candiasis in one patient [32].

Four studies have reported the efficacy of VSL#3 probiotic as maintenance therapy, the two RCTs both reported a remission rate at 6 months and 1 year respectively of 85%. However subsequent reports from real-world clinical practice at the

Cleveland clinic and St. Mark's hospital reported remission rates of 20% and 13% respectively [19]. These differences may in part be explained by careful selection of individuals including recruiting only those patients who achieved complete mucosal healing following antibiotic therapy.

An algorithm for the treatment of pouchitis is shown in Fig. 9.1.

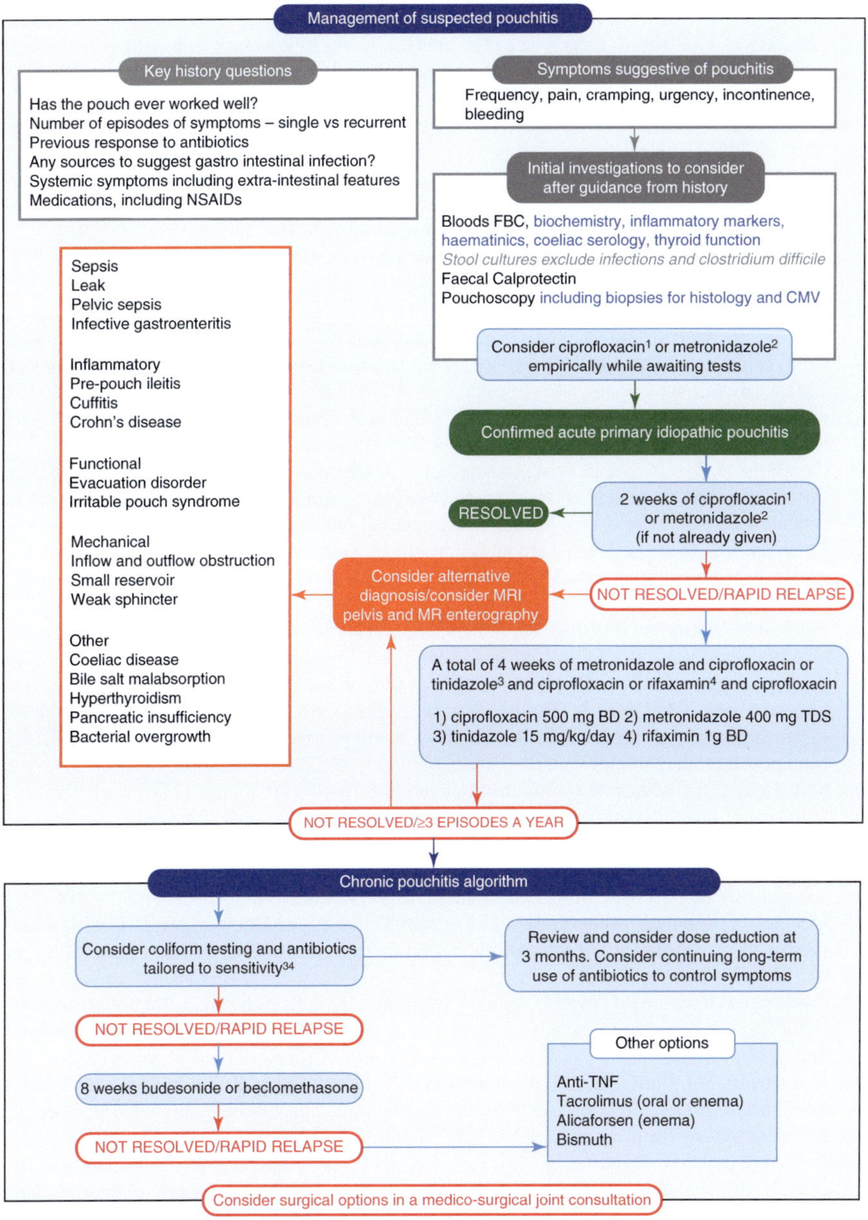


**Fig. 9.1** Algorithm for the treatment of pouchitis

## References

1. Romanos J, Samarasekera DN, Stebbing JF, Jewell DP, Kettlewell MG, Mortensen NJ. Outcome of 200 restorative proctocolectomy operations: the John Radcliffe Hospital experience. Br J Surg. 1997;84(6):814–8.
2. Hahnloser D, Pemberton JH, Wolff BG, Larson DR, Crownhart BS, Dozois RR. Results at up to 20 years after ileal pouch-anal anastomosis for chronic ulcerative colitis. Br J Surg. 2007;94(3):333–40.
3. Ståhlberg D, Gullberg K, Liljeqvist L, Hellers G, Löfberg R. Pouchitis following pelvic pouch operation for ulcerative colitis. Incidence, cumulative risk, and risk factors. Dis Colon Rectum. 1996;39(9):1012–8.
4. Sartor RB. Microbial influences in inflammatory bowel diseases. Gastroenterology. 2008;134(2):577–94.
5. Frank DN, St Amand AL, Feldman RA, Boedeker EC, Harpaz N, Pace NR. Molecular-phylogenetic characterization of microbial community imbalances in human inflammatory bowel diseases. Proc Natl Acad Sci U S A. 2007;104(34):13780–5.
6. Eckburg PB, Relman DA. The role of microbes in Crohn's disease. Clin Infect Dis. 2007;44(2):256–62.
7. Falk A, Olsson C, Ahrné S, Molin G, Adawi D, Jeppsson B. Ileal pelvic pouch microbiota from two former ulcerative colitis patients, analysed by DNA-based methods, were unstable over time and showed the presence of Clostridium perfringens. Scand J Gastroenterol. 2007;42(8):973–85.
8. Kühbacher T, Ott SJ, Helwig U, Mimura T, Rizzello F, Kleessen B, et al. Bacterial and fungal microbiota in relation to probiotic therapy (VSL#3) in pouchitis. Gut. 2006;55(6):833–41.
9. Casadesus D, Tani T, Wakai T, Maruyama S, Iiai T, Okamoto H, et al. Possible role of human cytomegalovirus in pouchitis after proctocolectomy with ileal pouch-anal anastomosis in patients with ulcerative colitis. World J Gastroenterol. 2007;13(7):1085–9.
10. Komanduri S, Gillevet PM, Sikaroodi M, Mutlu E, Keshavarzian A. Dysbiosis in pouchitis: evidence of unique microfloral patterns in pouch inflammation. Clin Gastroenterol Hepatol. 2007;5(3):352–60.
11. Johnson MW, Rogers GB, Bruce KD, Lilley AK, von Herbay A, Forbes A, et al. Bacterial community diversity in cultures derived from healthy and inflamed ileal pouches after restorative proctocolectomy. Inflamm Bowel Dis. 2009;15(12):1803–11.
12. Lim M, Adams JD, Wilcox M, Finan P, Sagar P, Burke D. An assessment of bacterial dysbiosis in pouchitis using terminal restriction fragment length polymorphisms of 16S ribosomal DNA from pouch effluent microbiota. Dis Colon Rectum. 2009;52(8):1492–500.
13. McLaughlin SD, Walker AW, Churcher C, Clark SK, Tekkis PP, Johnson MW, et al. The bacteriology of pouchitis: a molecular phylogenetic analysis using 16S rRNA gene cloning and sequencing. Ann Surg. 2010;252(1):90–8.
14. Reshef L, Kovacs A, Ofer A, Yahav L, Maharshak N, Keren N, et al. Pouch inflammation is associated with a decrease in specific bacterial taxa. Gastroenterology. 2015;149(3):718–27.
15. Machiels K, Sabino J, Vandermosten L, Joossens M, Arijs I, de Bruyn M, et al. Specific members of the predominant gut microbiota predict pouchitis following colectomy and IPAA in UC. Gut. 2017;66(1):79–88.
16. Gionchetti P, Rizzello F, Helwig U, Venturi A, Lammers KM, Brigidi P, et al. Prophylaxis of pouchitis onset with probiotic therapy: a double-blind, placebo-controlled trial. Gastroenterology. 2003;124(5):1202–9.
17. McLaughlin SD, Clark SK, Bell AJ, Tekkis PP, Ciclitira PJ, Nicholls RJ. Incidence and short-term implications of prepouch ileitis following restorative proctocolectomy with ileal pouch-anal anastomosis for ulcerative colitis. Dis Colon Rectum. 2009;52(5):879–83.
18. Bell AJ, Price AB, Forbes A, Ciclitira PJ, Groves C, Nicholls RJ. Pre-pouch ileitis: a disease of the ileum in ulcerative colitis after restorative proctocolectomy. Colorectal Dis. 2006;8(5):402–10.

19. Segal JP, Ding NS, Worley G, Mclaughlin S, Preston S, Faiz OD, et al. Systematic review with meta-analysis: the management of chronic refractory pouchitis with an evidence-based treatment algorithm. Aliment Pharmacol Ther. 2017;45(5):581–92.
20. Gionchetti P, Calabrese C, Calafiore A, Praticò C, Poggioli G, Laureti S, et al. Oral beclomethasone dipropionate in chronic refractory pouchitis. J Crohns Colitis. 2014;8(7):649–53.
21. Belluzzi A, Serrani M, Roda G, Bianchi ML, Castellani L, Grazia M, et al. Pilot study: the use of sulfasalazine for the treatment of acute pouchitis. Aliment Pharmacol Ther. 2010;31(2):228–32.
22. Uchino M, Ikeuchi H, Bando T, Matsuoka H, Hirata A, Takahashi Y, et al. Diffuse gastroduodenitis and enteritis associated with ulcerative colitis and concomitant cytomegalovirus reactivation after total colectomy: report of a case. Surg Today. 2013;43(3):321–4.
23. Greuter T, Biedermann L, Rogler G, Sauter B, Seibold F. Alicaforsen, an antisense inhibitor of ICAM-1, as treatment for chronic refractory pouchitis after proctocolectomy: a case series. United European Gastroenterol J. 2016;4(1):97–104.
24. Zins BJ, Sandborn WJ, Penna CR, Landers CJ, Targan SR, Tremaine WJ, et al. Pouchitis disease course after orthotopic liver transplantation in patients with primary sclerosing cholangitis and an ileal pouch-anal anastomosis. Am J Gastroenterol. 1995;90(12):2177–81.
25. Rowley S, Candinas D, Mayer AD, Buckels JA, McMaster P, Keighley MR. Restorative proctocolectomy and pouch anal anastomosis for ulcerative colitis following orthotopic liver transplantation. Gut. 1995;37(6):845–7.
26. Tremaine WJ, Sandborn WJ, Wolff BG, Carpenter HA, Zinsmeister AR, Metzger PP. Bismuth carbomer foam enemas for active chronic pouchitis: a randomized, double-blind, placebo-controlled trial. Aliment Pharmacol Ther. 1997;11(6):1041–6.
27. McLaughlin SD, Culkin A, Cole J, Clark SK, Tekkis PP, Ciclitira PJ, et al. Exclusive elemental diet impacts on the gastrointestinal microbiota and improves symptoms in patients with chronic pouchitis. J Crohns Colitis. 2013;7(6):460–6.
28. Landy J, Walker AW, Li JV, Al-Hassi HO, Ronde E, English NR, et al. Variable alterations of the microbiota, without metabolic or immunological change, following faecal microbiota transplantation in patients with chronic pouchitis. Sci Rep. 2015;5:12955.
29. McLaughlin SD, Clark SK, Bell AJ, Tekkis PP, Ciclitira PJ, Nicholls RJ. An open study of antibiotics for the treatment of pre-pouch ileitis following restorative proctocolectomy with ileal pouch-anal anastomosis. Aliment Pharmacol Ther. 2009;29(1):69–74.
30. Calabrese C, Gionchetti P, Rizzello F, Liguori G, Gabusi V, Tambasco R, et al. Short-term treatment with infliximab in chronic refractory pouchitis and ileitis. Aliment Pharmacol Ther. 2008;27(9):759–64.
31. McLaughlin SD, Clark SK, Tekkis PP, Ciclitira PJ, Nicholls RJ. Review article: restorative proctocolectomy, indications, management of complications and follow-up--a guide for gastroenterologists. Aliment Pharmacol Ther. 2008;27(10):895–909.
32. McLaughlin SD, Clark SK, Tekkis PP, Ciclitira PJ, Nicholls RJ. An open study of maintenance antibiotic therapy for chronic antibiotic-dependent pouchitis: efficacy, complications and outcome. Colorectal Dis. 2011;13(4):438–44.

# Chapter 10
# Ileoanal Pouch for Familial Adenomatous Polyposis

**Ashish Sinha and Sue Clark**

**Abstract** Formation of an ileoanal pouch, either at initial large bowel surgery to manage familial adenomatous polyposis, or if the rectum requires removal following previous colectomy with ileorectal anastomosis, is a very useful surgical option. It permits removal of virtually all large bowel mucosa, and hence colorectal cancer risk. It is not, however a panacea, and seems to be associated with increased desmoid formation, as well as neoplasia of the small bowel mucosa of the pouch. Careful counselling by a medical team fully conversant with these issues is essential before offering a patient such surgery.

**Keywords** Familial adenomatous polyposis · Prophylactic surgery · Ileoanal pouch · Restorative proctocolectomy · Desmoid

## 10.1 Familial Adenomatous Polyposis

Familial adenomatous polyposis (FAP) is an inherited colorectal cancer predisposition syndrome with population prevalence between 1 in 7500 and 1 in 13,000 [1, 2], accounting for less than 1% of all new colorectal cancer diagnoses in the United Kingdom.

## 10.2 The Genotype

FAP is inherited in an autosomal dominant fashion, with very high penetrance, meaning that virtually all individuals with FAP develop the defining feature of over 100 colorectal adenomas with inevitable progression to colorectal cancer in the

A. Sinha · S. Clark (✉)
The Polyposis Registry, St. Mark's Hospital, London North West University Healthcare NHS Trust, Harrow, UK

Department of Surgery and Cancer, Imperial College, London, UK
e-mail: s.clark8@nhs.net



J. Warusavitarne, Z. Perry-Woodford (eds.), *The Ileoanal Pouch*,
https://doi.org/10.1007/978-3-319-94385-5_10

absence of surgical intervention [1]. It is caused by inheritance of a mutation in one copy the adenomatous polyposis coli (*APC*) tumour suppressor gene (the germline mutation), with the phenotype developing when the single remaining normal (wild-type) copy is lost in a cell by somatic mutation. A quarter of all cases are thought to arise by *de novo* germline mutation, which occurs during reproduction rather than being inherited [1, 3].

The *APC* gene is large; it consists of 21 exons within a 98kB locus, of which 16 exons are translated into a 2861 amino acid protein. Exon 15 predominates, contributing in excess of 75% of the total coding sequence and is the region in which the majority of germline and somatic mutations occur.

*APC* is expressed very broadly, and the protein product plays a key role in the Wnt signalling pathway, which is deranged in the early stages of formation of most colorectal adenomas [4]. This pathway is also important in development and growth of three-dimensional structures throughout the body.

### *10.2.1 Other Adenomatous Polyposis Syndromes*

More recently, mutations in the *MutYH* gene have been found to cause a recessively inherited form of adenomatous polyposis (*MutYH* associated polyposis [MAP]), with generally later onset and fewer adenomas than FAP, but considerable phenotypic overlap [5]. Dominantly acting mutation of the DNA polymerase proofreading genes *POLE* or *POLD1* has also been found to result in an attenuated form of adenomatous polyposis (polymerase proofreading associated polyposis [PPAP]) [6].

## 10.3 Clinical Manifestations

The ubiquitous expression and broad function of the *APC* gene makes FAP a truly multi-system disorder. In patients who have undergone prophylactic colectomy, effectively preventing colorectal cancer, duodenal cancer and desmoid are the leading causes of death [7, 8].

### *10.3.1 The Gastrointestinal Tract*

FAP predisposes to the development of hundreds to thousands of adenomatous polyps in the large bowel, which are usually present by early adolescence. If these adenomas are not removed, carcinoma develops by the end of fourth decade of life in the vast majority [7].

FAP can also involve other parts of the gastrointestinal tract, especially the stomach and duodenum. Most of the gastric lesions seen in FAP patients are fundic gland polyps with no malignant potential. However 90% of patients with FAP develop duodenal adenomas, particularly in the ampullary region. A minority (about 10%)

progress to invasive carcinoma, which is associated with an extremely poor prognosis and tends to occur at a later age than colorectal carcinoma [9].

Surveillance of the upper gastrointestinal tract is carried out from age 25 years using end and side viewing duodenoscopy. Surveillance intervals are guided by the Spigelman stage, incorporating polyp number, size, histology and extent of dysplasia [2]. Patients with stage IV duodenal polyposis are at 36% risk of developing an invasive carcinoma within the next 10 years [9]; some patients undergo prophylactic duodenectomy to prevent this.

### *10.3.2 Desmoid Disease*

Desmoids are rare myofibroblastic proliferations that typically occur along musculo-aponeurotic planes and in the small bowel mesentery. Only about 10% of desmoids are found in association with FAP, where they occur in 10–20% of individuals. They are about four times more common in those with germline mutation in a particular region of the *APC* gene; family history of desmoid, independent of the germline mutation site (presumably due to a modifier gene [10]), increases the risk even more markedly (up to seven-fold) and female gender is also a risk factor. Desmoid formation appears to be triggered by trauma, which often takes the form of surgery [11].

Small bowel mesenteric desmoid is thought to start as small plaques of mesenteric fibromatosis, which can become more diffuse in some patients. This can often be asymptomatic and go undetected, but can render further surgery technically difficult. Only a small proportion progress further to form a frank desmoid mass. The vast majority cease growth spontaneously, and only 10–20% grow relentlessly. Whilst they do not metastasise, they can be locally invasive and cause complications by obstructing the ureters and bowel. This minority, however, is an important cause of severe morbidity and mortality in patients with FAP.

### *10.3.3 Other Cancers*

Carcinomas in other organs including the thyroid, gallbladder, pancreas, and adrenal gland are all associated with FAP, and hepatoblastoma and medulloblastoma also occur with increased incidence [2].

### *10.3.4 Benign Extra-Colonic Manifestations*

Benign extra-colonic manifestations seen in FAP include isolated or multiple osteomas of the skull and mandible, epidermoid cysts of the skin and dental anomalies. Congenital hypertrophy of the retinal pigment epithelium (CHRPE) is a harmless patchy hamartomatous retinal pigmentation frequently encountered in patients with FAP.

### *10.3.5 Genotype-Phenotype Correlation in FAP*

There are several established relationships between the site of *APC* mutation and the clinical manifestations of disease that results (Nieuwenhuis 2007); understanding of these is important in managing patients with FAP.

Patients with an *APC* mutation around codon 1309 (1300–1315) have an exceptionally severe colorectal phenotype. These individuals have a high colorectal adenoma burden (usually more than a thousand polyps), develop colorectal cancer at an early age, and are at high risk of progressive disease in the retained rectum if a colectomy with ileorectal anastomosis is performed [12].

The 'mutation cluster region' (MCR) corresponds to the area between codons 1250 and 1450 on exon 15 of the *APC* gene, and is a common site of germline mutation. Mutation in this region is associated with 'classical' polyposis, usually with several hundred colorectal adenomas.

Germline mutations 5′ of codon 160 and 3′ of codon 1450 are associated with an attenuated phenotype, with later onset of more scanty adenomas (often fewer than 100). A four-fold increased predisposition to desmoid development is described in patients with mutation 3′ to codon 1399 [11].

## 10.4 Clinical Management of FAP

### *10.4.1 Surveillance and Diagnosis*

About 75% of patients with FAP have inherited the condition from one or other parent. Improvements in genetic services and cascade testing mean that the vast majority of these individuals are known to be at-risk, and undergo appropriate surveillance. This can fail due to factors including adoption, non-paternity, absence of appropriate referral of FAP cases, or lack of engagement with healthcare providers. These individuals, and those with *de novo* mutation, present symptomatically with large adenomas or even invasive cancer.

If the germline *APC* mutation causing FAP in a family is known, predictive genetic testing will be available for at-risk family members, and is usually performed around that age of 12 years. It is unusual to develop extensive symptomatic adenomas or severe dysplasia earlier, although this can occur (particularly in association with mutation in codon 1309 of the *APC* gene). If an at-risk child develops anaemia, chronic diarrhoea or rectal bleeding, testing should be done promptly. In 10–15% of families with a classical phenotype of FAP (over 100 adenomas) no *APC* mutation can be detected. At-risk individuals in such families are surveyed by flexible sigmoidoscopy or colonoscopy.

Once the diagnosis of FAP has been confirmed in an at-risk individual, a colonoscopy is performed specifically to assess their colonic and rectal adenoma burden. If they are over 25 years of age, upper gastrointestinal endoscopy should also be performed.

The large bowel adenomas in FAP are too numerous and widespread to manage endoscopically, except in rare truly attenuated cases. Current strategies for managing FAP focus around the need for prophylactic colectomy prior to the onset of invasive cancer, an approach strongly supported by markedly improved survival when this is adopted [13]. The main decisions needed address the timing and type of prophylactic surgery.

## 10.5 Timing of Surgery in FAP

Modern surgical management of FAP aims to offer prophylactic surgery, well before colorectal cancer develops. To achieve this, screen-detected patients usually undergo surgery in their late teens or early twenties. The authors' preference is to undertake surgery in those from 'classical' FAP families during the summer vacation when they are 16 years old. This occurs after major public examinations, when there is a period of several weeks of holiday. This allows time for recovery and creates minimal social and educational disruption. Most young people of this age are still living with their parents, which facilitates attendance and ensures care and support at home during the recovery period. The patients are almost fully grown, facilitating surgery by adult colorectal surgeons familiar with FAP, and are also sufficiently mature to take an active part in the decision making process.

Occasionally, younger children present symptomatically and with a significant adenoma burden, and surgery is needed earlier. Some patients do not present until later, in which cases urgency is determined by the presence of frank invasive malignancy or concerning polyps.

A few patients have a genuinely attenuated phenotype, and can be safely managed endoscopically for many years, although this is applies to a very small proportion with FAP. A greater proportion of individuals with MAP or PPAP can be managed without surgery until much later into adult life.

One other rationale for delaying surgery is to reduce the risk of desmoid, which is frequently triggered by surgical trauma. There is some evidence [14] to support this in individuals at high risk of desmoid. These are people who already have a diagnosis of desmoid before undergoing prophylactic surgery, those with a strong family history of desmoid, and those with a germline *APC* mutation predictive of a high risk of desmoid (3′ of codon 1399) [11]. This latter group often have an attenuated colorectal phenotype, allowing prophylactic surgery to be safely delayed for quite some time.

## 10.6 Surgical Options

The choice of surgery lies between colectomy with ileorectal anastomosis (IRA), restorative proctocolectomy (RPC) with formation of an ileoanal pouch, or total proctocolectomy with end ileostomy (TPC). There is no place for segmental colectomy, even when adenomas appear predominantly in one region, as the risk of developing adenomas in the residual large bowel is extremely high.

Prior to the mid-nineteenth century, the risks associated with extensive large bowel surgery precluded its use prophylactically. With the advent of safer anaesthetics, antibiotics and sound anastomotic technique, IRA became established in the 1950s. It was the preferred prophylactic technique, as the permanent ileostomy associated with TPC was avoided.

Total proctocolectomy is extremely effective in preventing colorectal cancer in FAP as it removes all large bowel mucosa. This is, however, at the cost of a permanent ileostomy and exposure to the risks of pelvic dissection. It is therefore rarely used prophylactically, but is necessary when a very low cancer or mesenteric desmoid precludes reconstructive surgery, or if a patient does not wish to undergo RPC.

Until the mid 1980s, follow-up after IRA was done using rigid sigmoidoscopy of the remaining rectum. Large adenomas were removed by fulguration under general anaesthetic, and completion proctectomy and formation of an ileostomy was sometimes necessary. There were a number of reports of high rates of cancer in the retained rectum as patients reached their 50s, which gave rise to some concern. Historical series suggested that 12–43% of patients developed cancer in the rectal remnant by 20 years after IRA, and in one series a third of patients had undergone completion proctectomy at a median follow-up of a little under 20 years following IRA [15]. However, these data originate from a time when IRA was performed for almost all cases of FAP, regardless of polyp density or phenotype (the ‘pre-pouch era’).

When RPC was introduced in the late 1970s, it appeared the obvious solution to the problem of the retained rectum, and was universally adopted in some institutions. Others, however, developed a selective policy, enabled by the advent of flexible endoscopy and discovery of the genetic basis of FAP at around the same time.

An understanding of genotype-phenotype correlation allows prediction of severe or mild large bowel disease, at least to some extent. Pre-operative colonoscopy provides an accurate estimation of adenoma burden in the colon and rectum, distinguishing mild and more severe phenotypes. In patients who have undergone IRA, flexible sigmoidoscopy and modern polypectomy techniques allow much improved management of the retained rectum. The option of formation of an ileoanal pouch in most cases if the retained rectum becomes endoscopically unmanageable makes completion proctectomy a much more palatable prospect when it becomes necessary than was previously the case.

## 10.7 The Place of Restorative Proctocolectomy as Primary Surgery for FAP

### *10.7.1 Patients with FAP and Rectal Cancer*

RPC should be considered in any patient with FAP (or another adenomatous polyposis syndrome) and rectal cancer that is not so low as to preclude sphincter-sparing surgery. Such individuals require oncological surgery for their rectal cancer, according to normal principles, and prophylactic removal of the remaining large bowel. The need for pre-operative radiotherapy is not a contra-indication to ileoanal pouch formation, as the terminal ileum that will be used to fashion the pouch is not in the radiation field.

### 10.7.2 Prophylactic Surgery

The aim of prophylactic surgery in FAP is to minimise large bowel cancer risk and surgical complications and at the same time provide good functional outcome and quality of life. Both IRA and RPC do this, but with a different balance of risk and benefit. It is important to note that the context of an otherwise healthy adolescent undergoing prophylactic surgery for future cancer prevention is very different from that of a patient with ulcerative colitis facing proctocolectomy to control active disease. Risks of complications and suboptimal function that might be acceptable in the latter group are not in the former [16], in whom expectations in terms of outcomes are much higher.

Studies [17] have shown that IRA is associated with better functional outcome (lower defaecatory frequency and faecal incontinence rate) and quality of life [18]. It spares these young patients the morbidity of a pelvic dissection and retains the native rectum. It has fewer complications, does not require temporary faecal diversion and is more acceptable to healthy adolescents undergoing prophylactic surgery.

Regular (6–12 monthly) flexible sigmoidoscopic follow-up is required, and as patients age, some go on to require completion proctectomy (at which it is usually possible to create an ileoanal pouch). That said, a large follow-up study has shown that around 50% of patients who had undergone IRA retained a healthy rectum at age 60, even though the cohort studied included all patients undergoing IRA, many from the 'pre-pouch era', pre-dating any form of selective surgery [19].

Ileoanal pouch surgery results in reduced female fertility [20] (a risk that might be lessened by performing the surgery using a laparoscopic approach), caries a small risk of erectile and ejaculatory dysfunction [21] and has the potential for a permanent ileostomy if pouch failure occurs. In the context of FAP this is far more likely to be due to septic complications than to primary idiopathic pouchitis, which can occur but is much less common than following surgery for ulcerative colitis. One large series has documented a 10% pouch failure rate in FAP patients on long-term follow-up [22].

The rationale behind a selective approach to surgery is that patients with relatively mild large bowel adenomatosis have a low risk of rectal cancer if they have good quality endoscopic follow-up following IRA, and to perform RPC in this group is 'overkill', exposing them to poorer function and increased complications for little gain.

Those with a more severe phenotype, or predicted to develop more severe disease because of the *APC* mutation they have inherited, are better served by undergoing RPC as their initial prophylactic surgery, despite the potential drawbacks. This approach avoids the need for further surgery after a short time, and the high risk of rectal cancer developing if the rectum affected by a high adenoma burden is not removed.

Several institutions have adopted this approach, which is now supported by good quality evidence [15, 19, 23, 24]. The criteria used to aid decision make have evolved, and those currently used by the St. Mark's Hospital Polyposis Registry are shown on Table 10.1. A study of the large Cleveland Clinic cohort [15] has shown a very marked reduction in the need for completion proctectomy following IRA after a selective policy has been adopted. A study from St. Mark's looked back at patients who had undergone IRA historically, and stratified eventual outcome according to various factors, including genotype. The survival curves shown in Fig. 10.1 illustrate the marked effect of mutation site on the likelihood of retaining a healthy rectum in the long term after IRA.

**Table 10.1** Criteria for recommending restorative proctocolectomy as prophylactic surgery for FAP

| Criteria |
|---|
| > 500 colonic polyps |
| OR |
| > 20 rectal polyps |
| OR |
| *APC* mutation between codons 1250 and 1450 |
| OR |
| Rectal adenoma not endocopically resectable |

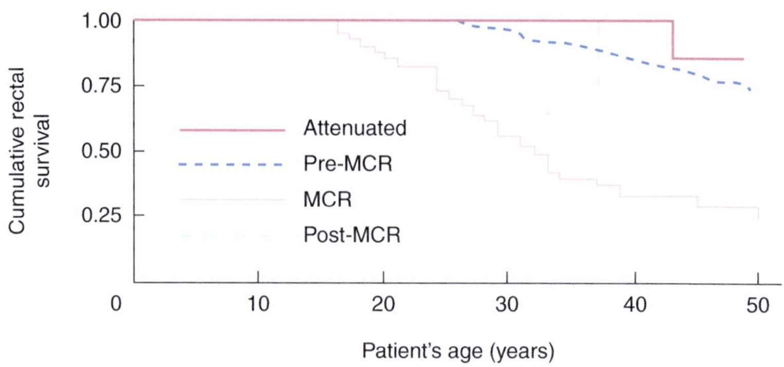


No. at risk

| | 0 | 10 | 20 | 30 | 40 | 50 |
|---|---|---|---|---|---|---|
| Attenuated | 28 | 28 | 27 | 22 | 16 | 9 |
| Pre-MCR | 228 | 225 | 205 | 157 | 102 | 52 |
| MCR | 44 | 44 | 35 | 18 | 9 | 6 |
| Post-MCR | 14 | 14 | 12 | 8 | 1 | 1 |

**Fig. 10.1** Rectal failure following ileorectal anastomosis in relation to patient age, stratified by *APC* mutation. (Attenuated, codons 1–159; pre-MCR, codons 160–1249; MCR, codons 1250–1450; post-MCR, 3′ of codon 1450). (Reproduced from Sinha et al. [19] with permission)

## 10.8 The Ileoanal Pouch in Secondary Surgery

Following IRA, patients require on going surveillance of the retained rectum. Typically, they undergo 6–12 monthly flexible sigmoidoscopy with endoscopic therapy to mange rectal polyposis. Eventually some require completion proctectomy, with or without restoration of continuity using an ileoanal pouch, either for worsening polyp burden or rectal cancer.

Most patients in this category will be in their 50s or older, and many have co-morbidities which impact on decision making. As all have a history of previous colectomy, it is sensible to perform cross-sectional imaging of the abdomen to look for evidence of small bowel mesenteric fibromatosis or frank desmoid mass, which might make ileal pouch construction or ileal pouch-anal anastomosis impossible. It is also important to ensure that duodenal surveillance is up to date before embarking upon major pelvic surgery.

Several series [22, 25, 26] have shown similar outcomes in patients undergoing formation of ileoanal pouch having had IRA previously as in those undergoing RPC as their primary operation. This supports the approach of offering this procedure as a 'second line' option in those who develop unmanageable adenomatosis of the retained rectum following IRA.

While the concept of a single operation to manage the large bowel in FAP is attractive, in practice this means exposing many healthy adolescents to potentially unnecessary pelvic surgery and stoma formation (albeit usually temporary). A selective approach to surgery will never be perfect, however, and some of those undergoing IRA will eventually need completion proctectomy, although the necessity for this after a short interval should be avoided. By that stage most will be in established employment and relationships, and have completed their family. They will be better equipped to face the risks of pelvic surgery, and the prospect of an ileostomy, whether temporary or permanent. There will also be less time in which an ileoanal pouch can itself develop neoplasia, as such individuals are around 35–40 years older than those undergoing initial prophylactic surgery for FAP.

## 10.9 Desmoid Disease and the Ileoanal Pouch

### *10.9.1 Surgery as a Stimulus to Desmoid Formation*

The majority of abdominal wall and intra-abdominal desmoids in FAP occur in the 2 years following prophylactic colectomy. It has been observed that performing colectomy at a young age is associated with increased risk of desmoid formation in females [14].

Some authors have shown an increased risk of desmoid following RPC compared with IRA [27] with a hazard ratio of 1.67. Other studies show no difference, but are limited by small size and varying selection criteria for surgery, with resulting

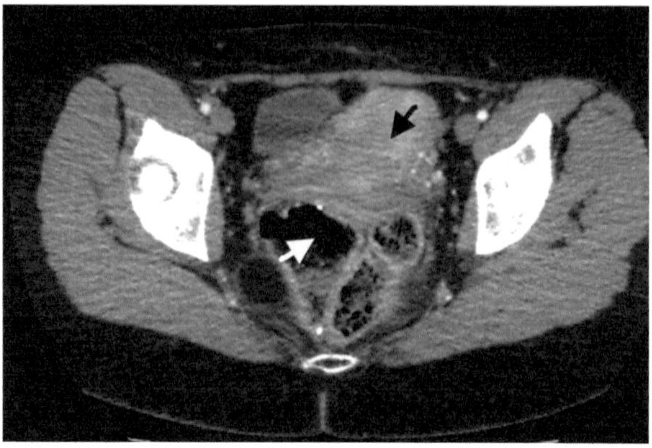

**Fig. 10.2** CT scan showing ileoanal pouch (lumen indicated by white arrow) with desmoid tumour of the associated mesentery (black arrow)

bias. Figure 10.2 shows a CT scan of a patient with FAP and an ileoanal pouch with desmoid tumour of the associated mesentery.

It might be expected that performing surgery laparoscopically would reduce desmoid formation, as abdominal wall trauma is less, and although essentially the same surgery is performed internally, there is less direct traction, cooling and drying of tissues. A recent study [27] demonstrated a reduction in post-operative desmoid tumour rate from 13% to 5% when a laparoscopic approach was adopted; the majority of the patients described underwent IRA. Data from the Cleveland Clinic are similar, with desmoid occurring in 3.8% after laparoscopically assisted IRA compared with 15.8% after open IRA [28].

There is some evidence that laparoscopically assisted RPC is associated with a particularly high risk of desmoid formation (46%). It is not clear why this should be so, and it has been suggested that increased tension in the ileal mesentery may be responsible [28].

Reassuringly, there does not appear to be any difference in morbidity if a patient develops desmoid disease after RPC compared with after IRA, suggesting that the presence of desmoid or high risk of desmoid should not be a contraindication to RPC [29].

### *10.9.2 Decision Making in 'Desmoid Prone' Patients*

'Desmoid prone' patients, who are at particularly high risk of developing problematic abdominal wall or intra-abdominal desmoids following prophylactic large bowel excision, are those with pre-existing desmoid disease, a family history of desmoid, or *APC* mutation 3′ of codon 1399; many such individuals will have more than one of these risk factors, and females appears to be more vulnerable [11, 30].

In this group it seems sensible to postpone prophylactic surgery as long as is feasible; quite a long delay is often possible as those with *APC* mutation 3′ of codon 1399 rather fortuitously also tend to have a more attenuated phenotype, with fewer colorectal adenomas of rather later onset than average.

Cross-sectional imaging to assess for the presence of sub-clinical desmoid is wise, and allows the patient and surgeon to be as fully informed as possible before surgery. Unexpected pre-existing desmoid was found in 3% of patients of patients undergoing colectomy for FAP in one large series [31], and is more likely in those with recognised risk factors.

In terms of which operation should be performed, some argue that RPC is preferred, because desmoid formation after IRA can render completion proctectomy impossible [2] - there is, however, only one case such as this reported, and the precise circumstances are unclear. The Cleveland Clinic group found no evidence of desmoid preventing proctectomy in their extensive practice [32]. On the other hand, performing RPC may me more likely to stimulate desmoid formation, and given the attenuated colorectal phenotype in many of these patients, proctectomy may never be necessary.

The practice at the authors' institution is to use the same criteria as outlined in Table 10.1 to guide the choice of surgery. If RPC is indicated, it is performed by open surgery when patients are at high risk of desmoid, but laparoscopically if they are not.

### *10.9.3 Pre-existing Desmoid*

Rarely, patients develop desmoid in childhood or adolescence, before undergoing any abdominal surgery. The presence of abdominal wall or intra-abdominal desmoid in such individuals can make colectomy or proctocolectomy extremely challenging. It may be impossible to form an ileal pouch, to get it to reach the anus, or to form a protective ileostomy above it. Most desmoid occurs after surgical trauma, usually prophylactic colectomy, and in a patient who already has desmoid, there is a high risk that surgery will stimulate further desmoid growth. Many such patients have a mild colorectal phenotype, and surgery should be deferred as long as appearances on annual colonoscopy are not concerning (no adenomas over 1 cm, no high grade dysplasia).

When the point is reached that prophylactic surgery can no longer be delayed, cross sectional imaging (CT or MRI) of the abdomen can be helpful in predicting the degree of difficulty of large bowel excision, and the likelihood of being able to form an ileoanal pouch.

## 10.10 Technical Controversies

### *10.10.1 Laparoscopic or Open Surgery?*

Most comparisons between open and laparoscopic RPC focus on the majority who undergo this surgery for ulcerative colitis and contain few, if any patients with FAP. However, in those where FAP is considered specifically [33, 34], there appears to be no difference other than the potential increase in risk of desmoid formation discussed above; laparoscopic RPC is associated with longer operating times, no excess of complications, similar functional outcomes and improved cosmesis compared with the same procedure performed open. Better cosmetic results and potential for less effect on fertility in females are particularly attractive features in this prophylactic setting.

### 10.10.2 Formation of the Ileal Pouch-Anal Anastomosis

When RPC was first performed, it was done using a mucosectomy and handsewn anastomosis. Later, the introduction of the circular stapler allowed the anastomosis to be formed more straightforwardly, and with better functional outcomes [35]. This is likely to be due to preservation of the ano-rectal transition zone, and its role in continence and defaecation, and avoidance of the anal dilatation required to perform a handsewn anastomosis.

The need for a mucosectomy to remove 'all' rectal mucosa prior to ileal pouch-anal anastomosis is still debated. Some argue that the risk of colorectal cancer is abolished since all at-risk mucosa is removed if a mucosectomy is performed prior to anastomosis. However, even what appears to be a complete mucosectomy can leave behind islands of rectal mucosa, which are then buried as the pouch is advanced. Indeed several cases of carcinoma arising at the anastomosis after mucosectomy have been reported, as well as after stapled anastomosis [36, 37]. Neither method therefore completely protects against cancer development at the anastomosis or rectal cuff.

While stapled anastomosis leaves the ano-rectal transition zone intact, the area remains straightforward to survey. Adenomas occur with greater frequency than after mucosectomy [38, 39] but these can easily and successfully be removed [38], although cancers have also been reported after stapled anastomosis [37, 40]. Such a cancer detected at routine follow-up is shown in Fig. 10.3.

The authors routinely perform stapled ileal pouch-anal anastomosis, leaving a cuff of no more than 1 cm in length above the dentate line, reserving mucosectomy and handsewn anastomosis for cases where extensive adenomas reach the dentate line.

## 10.11 Follow-Up After RPC in FAP

When RPC was first performed for FAP it was thought that it would abolish the need for regular endoscopic follow-up. However, the remaining small amount of rectal mucosa retained, even after mucosectomy, means that this region needs regular inspection, with removal of adenomas as they occur.

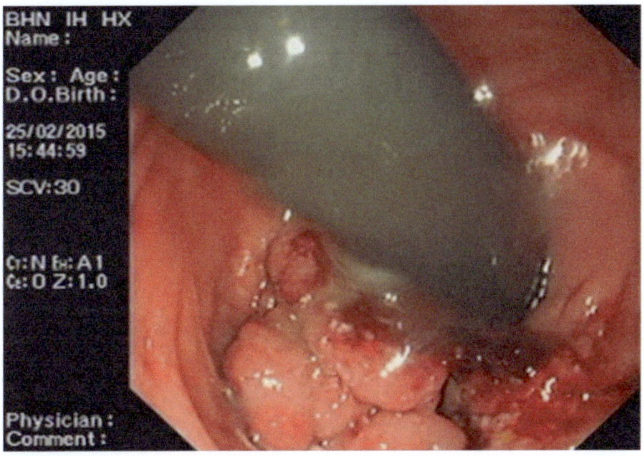


**Fig. 10.3** View with flexible scope in retroflexion showing carcinoma arising from the rectal cuff following stapled ileal pouch-anal anastomosis

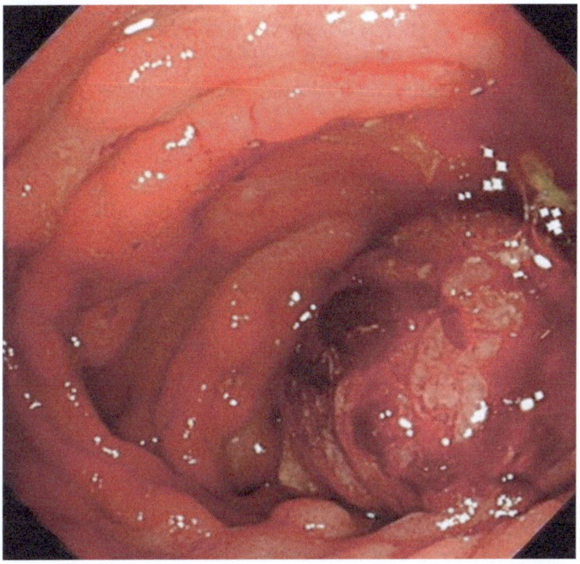

**Fig. 10.4** Flexible pouchoscopy showing adenomas of the ileal pouch body following RPC

It has now also become clear that the small bowel mucosa of the pouch body can also develop adenomas (Fig. 10.4), and even cancer. Ileal adenomas and carcinomas do occur in FAP, but are unusual. It seems that a change in environment, perhaps related to altered faecal microbiota, results in neoplasia becoming more frequent. This phenomenon has been observed in ileostomies, the ileum above IRA, and in the ileoanal pouch [41]. The majority (over 80% at 20 years) of ileoanal pouches do develop adenomas over time [42], with some reports of progression to cancer of the pouch body [43]. The strongest relationship is with age of the pouch, although there is some suggestion of correlation with severe duodenal adenoma formation [44].

Annual flexible pouchoscopy is recommended, and concern regarding neoplasia is now becoming an important indication for ileal pouch excision in patients with

FAP, though there is little on which to base risk prediction. This provides another argument for performing IRA when possible as primary prophylaxis, and keeping ileoanal pouch formation in reserve in case proctectomy is indicated later. Even avoiding pouch formation for 20–25 years may reduce the need for future pouch excision significantly [45].

## 10.12 Summary

The advent of the 'pouch era' coincided with identification of the *APC* gene and recognition of genotype-phenotype correlations in FAP. At the same time flexible endoscopy has allowed pre-operative stratification of severity of large bowel polyposis and better management of the retained rectum after IRA; the historical literature should be interpreted in the light of all of these developments.

Restorative proctocolectomy with formation of ileoanal pouch undoubtedly has a place in the management of FAP. Refinement of selection criteria and improved evidence based decision making now support the use of RPC as primary surgery only in more aggressive cases of FAP. The more stringent requirements of prophylactic surgery in healthy young people, and increasing evidence of ileal pouch neoplasia arising as the pouch ages, makes it unsuitable as the 'default' operation in FAP.

Careful selection of patients with a relatively mild phenotype, and without a genotype predictive of future severe disease, allows such individuals to be offered IRA with a good prospect of retaining a healthy rectum for most, if not all, of their life. Completion proctectomy with ileoanal pouch formation offers a sphincter-sparing solution for the vast majority of those who do eventually need to have their rectum removed.

For those with predictors of more aggressive large bowel polyposis, who are more likely to require subsequent proctectomy, undergoing RPC as their primary prophylactic procedure is likely to be the best option.

It is important to be mindful of the complex interrelationship between pouch surgery and desmoid disease, and to ensure that all patients with FAP and an ileoanal pouch undergo annual inspection of pouch (the anastomotic area and the pouch body) to identify early neoplasia.

## References


1. Bisgaard ML, Fenger K, Bulow S, Niebuhr E, Mohr J. Familial adenomatous polyposis (FAP): frequency, penetrance, and mutation rate. Hum Mutat. 1994;3:121–5.
2. Vasen HFA, Moslein G, Alonso A, et al. Guidelines for the clinical management of familial adenomatous polyposis (FAP). Gut. 2008;57:704–13.
3. Aretz S, Uhlhaas S, Caspari R, et al. Frequency and parental origin of de novo APC mutations in familial adenomatous polyposis. Eur J Hum Genet. 2004;12:52–8.
4. Chung DC. The genetic basis of colorectal cancer: insights into critical pathways of tumorigenesis. Gastroenterology. 2000;119:854–65.

5. Nielsen M, Morreau H, Vasen HF, et al. MUTYH-associated polyposis (MAP). Crit Rev Oncol Hematol. 2011;79:1–16.
6. Valle L, Hernández-Illán E, Bellido F, et al. New insights into POLE and POLD1 germline mutations in familial colorectal cancer and polyposis. Hum Mol Genet. 2014;23:3506–12.
7. Arvanitis ML, Jagelman DG, Fazio VW, Lavery IC, McGannon E. Mortality in patients with familial adenomatous polyposis. Dis Colon Rectum. 1990;33:639–42.
8. Gibbons DC, Sinha A, Phillips RK, et al. Colorectal cancer: no longer the issue in familial adenomatous polyposis? Fam Cancer. 2011;10:11–20.
9. Groves CJ, Saunders BP, Spigelman AD, et al. Duodenal cancer in patients with familial adenomatous polyposis (FAP): results of a 10 year prospective study. Gut. 2002;50:636–41.
10. Sturt NJ, Gallagher MC, Bassett P, et al. Evidence for genetic predisposition to desmoid tumours in familial adenomatous polyposis independent of the germline APC mutation. Gut. 2004;53:1832–6.
11. Sinha A, Tekkis PP, Neale KF, Phillips RKS, Clark SK. Risk factors predicting intra-abdominal desmoids in familial adenomatous polyposis: a single centre experience. Tech Coloproctol. 2010;14:141–6.
12. Nieuwenhuis MH, Vasen HF. Correlations between mutation site in APC and phenotype of familial adenomatous polyposis (FAP): a review of the literature. Crit Rev Oncol Hematol. 2007;61:153–61.
13. Koskenvuo L, Pitkaniemi J, Rantanen M, Lepisto A. Impact of screening on survival in familial adenomatous polyposis. J Clin Gastroenterol. 2016;50:40–4.
14. Durno C, Monga N, Bapat B, Berk T, Cohen Z, Gallinger S. Does early colectomy increase desmoid risk in familial adenomatous polyposis? Clin Gastroenterol Hepatol. 2007;5:1190–4.
15. Church J, Burke C, McGannon E, Pastean O, Clark B. Risk of rectal cancer in patients after colectomy and ileorectal anastomosis for familial adenomatous polyposis: a function of available surgical options. Dis Colon Rectum. 2003;46:1175–81.
16. Brennan MF. Pre-emptive surgery and increasing demands for technical perfection. Br J Surg. 2003;90:3–4.
17. Aziz O, Athanasiou T, Fazio VW, et al. Meta-analysis of observational studies of ileorectal versus ileal pouch-anal anastomosis for familial adenomatous polyposis. Br J Surg. 2006;93:407–17.
18. Gunther K, Braunrieder G, Bittorf BR, Hohenberger W, Matzel KE. Patients with familial adenomatous polyposis experience better bowel function and quality of life after ileorectal anastomosis than after ileoanal pouch. Colorectal Dis. 2003;5:38–44.
19. Sinha A, Tekkis PP, Rashid S, Phillips RKS, Clark SK. Risk factors for secondary proctectomy in patients with familial adenomatous polyposis. Br J Surg. 2010;97:1710–5.
20. Olsen K, Juul S, Bülow S, et al. Female fecundity before and after operation for familial adenomatous polyposis. Br J Surg. 2003;90:227–31.
21. Slors FJ, van Zuijlen PP, van Dijk GJ. Sexual and bladder dysfunction after total mesorectal excision for benign diseases. Scand J Gastroenterol Suppl. 2000:48–51.
22. von Roon AC, Tekkis PP, Lovegrove RE, Neale KF, Phillips RK, Clark SK. Comparison of outcomes of ileal pouch–anal anastomosis for familial adenomatous polyposis with and without previous ileorectal anastomosis. Br J Surg. 2008;95:494–8.
23. Bulow C, Vasen H, Jarvinen H, Bjork J, Bisgaard ML, Bulow S. Ileorectal anastomosis is appropriate for a subset of patients with familial adenomatous polyposis. Gastroenterology. 2000;119:1454–60.
24. Nieuwenhuis MH, Bulow S, Bjork J, et al. Genotype predicting phenotype in familial adenomatous polyposis: a practical application to the choice of surgery. Dis Colon Rectum. 2009;52:1259–63.
25. Penna C, Kartheuser A, Parc R, Tiret E, Frileux P, Hannoun L, et al. Secondary proctectomy and ileal pouch – anal anastomosis after ileorectal anastomosis familial adenomatous polyposis. Br J Surg. 1993;80:1621–3.
26. Bjork J, Akerbrant H, Iselius L, Svenberg T, Oresland T, Pahlman L, et al. Outcome of primary and secondary ileal pouch – anal anastomosis and ileorectal anastomosis in patients with familial adenomatous polyposis. Dis Colon Rectum. 2001;44:984–92.

27. Vitellaro M, Sala P, Signoroni S, et al. Risk of desmoid tumours after open and laparoscopic colectomy in patients with familial adenomatous polyposis. Br J Surg. 2014;101:558–65.
28. Vogel JD, Church JM, LaGuardia L. Minimally invasive pouch surgery predisposes to desmoid tumor formation in patients with familial adenomatous polyposis. Dis Colon Rectum. 2005;48:662–3.
29. Burgess A, Xhaja X, Church J. Does intra-abdominal desmoid disease affect patients with an ileal pouch differently than those with an ileorectal anastomosis? Dis Colon Rectum. 2011;54:1388–91.
30. Elayi E, Manilich E, Church J. Polishing the crystal ball: knowing genotype improves ability to predict desmoid disease in patients with familial adenomatous polyposis. Dis Colon Rectum. 2009;52:1762–6.
31. Hartley JE, Church JM, Gupta S, McGannon E, Fazio VW. Significance of incidental desmoids identified during surgery for familial adenomatous polyposis. Dis Colon Rectum. 2004;47:334–8.
32. Church JM, Xhaja X, Warrier SK, et al. Desmoid tumors do not prevent proctectomy following abdominal colectomy and ileorectal anastomosis in patients with familial adenomatous polyposis. Dis Colon Rectum. 2014;57:343–7.
33. Vitellaro M, Bonfanti G, Sala P, et al. Laparoscopic colectomy and restorative proctocolectomy for familial adenomatous polyposis. Surg Endosc. 2010;25:1866–75.
34. Ahmed Ali U, Keus F, Heikens JT, et al. Open versus laparoscopic (assisted) ileo pouch anal anastomosis for ulcerative colitis and familial adenomatous polyposis. Cochrane Database Syst Rev. 2009:CD006267.
35. Remzi FH, Church JM, Bast J, et al. Mucosectomy vs. stapled ileal pouch-anal anastomosis in patients with familial adenomatous polyposis: functional outcome and neoplasia control. Dis Colon Rectum. 2001;44:1590–6.
36. Brown SR, Donati D, Seow-Choen F. Rectal cancer after mucosectomy for ileoanal pouch in familial adenomatous polyposis: report of a case. Dis Colon Rectum. 2001;44:1714–5.
37. Ooi BS, Remzi FH, Gramlich T, Church JM, Preen M, Fazio VW. Anal transitional zone cancer after restorative proctocolectomy and ileoanal anastomosis in familial adenomatous polyposis: report of two cases. Dis Colon Rectum. 2003;46:1418–23.
38. von Roon AC, Will OC, Man RF, et al. Mucosectomy with handsewn anastomosis reduces the risk of adenoma formation in the anorectal segment after restorative proctocolectomy for familial adenomatous polyposis. Ann Surg. 2011;253:314–7.
39. Wasmuth HH, Tranø G, Myrvold HE, Aabakken L, Bakka A. Adenoma formation and malignancy after restorative proctocolectomy with or without mucosectomy in patients with familial adenomatous polyposis. Dis Colon Rectum. 2013;56:288–94.
40. Campos FG, Habr-Gama A, Kiss DR, et al. Adenocarcinoma after ileoanal anastomosis for familial adenomatous polyposis: review of risk factors and current surveillance apropos of a case. J Gastrointest Surg. 2005;9:695–702.
41. Groves CJ, Beveridge G, Swain DJ, et al. Prevalence and morphology of pouch and ileal adenomas in familial adenomatous polyposis. Dis Colon Rectum. 2005;48:816–23.
42. Will O, von Roon AC, Man RF, Neale KF, Tekkis PP, Clark SK. Long-term risk of pouch neoplasia after ileal pouch anal anastomosis for familial adenomatous polyposis. Hereditary Cancers Clin Pract. 2007;5:217.
43. Tajika M, Nakamura T, Nakahara O, et al. Prevalence of adenomas and carcinomas in the ileal pouch after proctocolectomy in patients with familial adenomatous polyposis. J Gastrointest Surg. 2009;13:1266–73.
44. Parc YR, Olschwang S, Desaint B, et al. Familial adenomatous polyposis: prevalence of adenomas in the ileal pouch after restorative proctocolectomy. Ann Surg. 2001;233:360–4.
45. Church J. Ileoanal pouch neoplasia in familial adenomatous polyposis: an underestimated threat. Dis Colon Rectum. 2005;48:1708–13.

# Chapter 11
# The Role of the Ileoanal Pouch Nurse Practitioner

**Zarah Perry-Woodford and Samantha Evans**

**Abstract** This chapter aims to illustrate the holistic approach undertaken by the pouch nurse practitioner (PNP) when imparting information, in order for patients to understand both the anatomical and psychological changes involved following restorative proctocolectomy (RPC) with ileal pouch anal anastomosis. The PNP is an advocate, mediating between the medical and surgical teams and is in an ideal position to assist in managing patient expectations of living with an ileoanal pouch. Advanced nursing skills are essential in supporting the patient to cope with a temporary ileostomy, altered bowel function and potential complications, in order to improve overall quality of life for those contemplating RPC.

**Keywords** Nurse-led care · Managing patient expectations · Complication management · Quality of life · Self-care · Stoma care · Counselling · Communication skills

## 11.1 Pre-operative Counselling

Restorative proctocolectomy (RPC) is a complex undertaking, requiring not only surgical expertise but extensive psychological and physical assessment in order to achieve satisfactory patient-reported outcomes. Appropriate patient selection and extensive pre-operative evaluation must be taken into consideration to prepare patients for this life changing operation [1]. RPC is not a return to 'normal' bowel function and the procedure carries significant risk and post-operative complications [2, 3]. Recent epidemiological studies suggest a higher rate of pan-colonic disease in South Asians compared to white Europeans [4], which presents not only cultural but communication barriers surrounding informed consent, patient understanding and overall nursing care.

Z. Perry-Woodford (✉) · S. Evans
St. Mark's Hospital, Harrow, UK
e-mail: zarah.perry-woodford@nhs.net



J. Warusavitarne, Z. Perry-Woodford (eds.), *The Ileoanal Pouch*,
https://doi.org/10.1007/978-3-319-94385-5_11

The majority of patients contemplating RPC have high expectations of surgery such as improved quality of life by avoiding a permanent ileostomy, alleviating the debilitating symptoms of ulcerative colitis (UC) or uncertainty of familial adenomatous polyposis (FAP), regaining physical and mental wellbeing, recouping lost opportunities due to periods of illness and reducing hospital visits and the potential to discontinue poly pharmacology [5]. Therefore it is paramount that individual patient expectations are fully understood by the pouch nurse practitioner (PNP) during the decision making process, as acceptable pouch function strongly correlates with high quality of life scores, in multiple domains of physical and psychosocial functioning [6]. RPC should be presented as an elective, multi-disciplinary decision with in-depth involvement from the patient, their family, medical team, surgical team and specialist nurses.

The aim of pre-operative counselling is not only to ensure the patient comprehends both the benefits and possible drawbacks of RPC but is made aware of suitable, alternative surgical options.

Pre-operative counselling should include:

- Information on normal bowel function and the influence of surgery on the gut
- Reiteration of the operative procedure and checking patient understanding
- Introduction to an enhanced recovery programme and post-operative care
- Brief discussion on laparoscopic vs open surgery
- Surgical options: RPC vs pan proctocolectomy and permanent ileostomy
- Patient suitability for RPC focusing on lifestyle, impact on work, education, hobbies, sport, travel and social life
- Patients expectations of living with a pouch/ileostomy
- Changes to body image and psychological support
- Sexual function changes
- Fertility, fecundity and pregnancy
- Stoma care- outlining differences between an end and loop ileostomy
- Demonstration with stoma starter kit and appliances
- Ileostomy (Stoma) siting
- Potential stoma complications and management
- Diet and fluid management
- Support groups/ networking
- Anal skin care
- Pouch complications including pouch failure
- Written information and PNP contact details
- Access to long term nurse-led advice

This is a vast amount of information to communicate and can be overwhelming for patients and their families, therefore it is important that counselling is staged according to the individual. Patients may be reviewed on multiple occasions pre-operatively to ensure they have understood the implications of surgery and to ensure appropriate candidate selection [1]. The main benefit of extensive pre-operative counselling and stoma education is to empower the patient, making them more responsive to the technicalities of stoma care or initial erratic pouch function [7]. Early and open communication also allows a therapeutic rapport to be established between the patient, surgeon and PNP.

**Table 11.1** Factors to consider prior to RPC

| Potential benefits | Considerations |
|---|---|
| Removal of disease<br>Eliminates the need for a permanent ileostomy<br>Patient choice<br>Improved body image and cosmesis<br>Increased sexual activity<br>Fewer dietary restrictions<br>Improved quality of life<br>Low risk to female fertility with laparoscopic approach | Multiple operations<br>Long operating times<br>Mainly performed at specialist centres<br>Financial implications for patient and family (travel time, appointments)<br>Uncertain outcomes<br>Inability to pass flatus spontaneously<br>Considerable time for pouch to settle into an acceptable routine<br>Pouch seepage at night or incontinence<br>Possible pouch complications<br>Reduced libido and sexual function associated with pouch dysfunction<br>Deterioration of function over time<br>Long-term hospital surveillance or follow up<br>Risk of pouch/cuff cancer<br>Pouch failure resulting in further operations and return to permanent ileostomy |

## 11.2 Factors to Consider Pre-operatively

The primary indication for RPC is to remove disease and avoid permanent ileostomy [8]. Though subjective, there are many factors which influence patients' decision making such as age, lifestyle, co- morbidities, personal experience and expectations of outcomes, support networks, family or peer pressure, fear of the unknown, knowledge and understanding of the operative procedures. Many of these factors are difficult for medical staff to comprehend, therefore it is essential that the PNP allows time for patients to balance personal perspectives and risk against medical statistics and data. Some patients benefit from discussing the lived experience with others who have undergone RPC. Table 11.1 lists the influencing factors to consider.

## 11.3 Sexuality and Sexual Function

Sexuality is a significant and often neglected subject in pre-operative counselling despite most patients facing RPC being young adults. Concerns regarding sexual relationships, fertility, conception and the ability to bear children must be addressed as young patients may still be developing their own sexuality and relationships [9, 10]. The physical and psychological effects of RPC impacts on the patients' readiness for intimacy, as lack of libido, fear of incontinence and dyspareunia during intercourse, may influence sexual behavior in both men and women [11, 12].

In men, damage to the pelvic autonomic nerves following RPC results in 4% erectile disorders and 3% ejaculatory disorders after 10 years [13]. Early sexual dysfunction commonly resolves spontaneously however lingering concerns should be addressed or referred for urological review. Thirty-six percent of patients reported reduced sexual activity or abstinence pre-operatively compared with 19% post-operatively, suggesting RPC improves sexual activity [13]. Sexual relationships should only be resumed when the patient feels ready and able to and when the surgical incisions have healed. Post operatively both men and women report improved body image, although there may be a tendency toward better body image among laparoscopy-treated women [14]. In women, there is a significant correlation between poor pouch function and impaired sexual function [9].

It is important that patients who engage in anal intercourse be counselled in depth by their surgeon and PNP on how RPC may impact on sexual relationships. Patients are advised to refrain from anal intercourse after RPC, as this practice can stretch and damage the sphincter muscles which can lead to incontinence and leakage [15]. If patients are concerned about completely refraining from anal intercourse, a hand-sewn instead of stapled anastomosis may be discussed with the surgeon to prevent staple injury to the partner. It is important for the PNP to be an advocate for the patient, to provide support in this vital aspect of sexuality and to assess for any difficulties for the patient or partner.

## 11.4 Fertility and Fecundity

The risk of infertility or sexual dysfunction should not preclude RPC as a suitable option especially for women of child bearing age. Twenty-four months following cessation of contraception, 67% of women had at least one pregnancy post RPC [16]. The same degree of risk to fertility and fecundity is associated with either RPC or pan-proctocolectomy as both procedures involve proctectomy (removal of the rectum). Proctectomy in women increases the risk of pelvic adhesions and tubal disruptions which may hinder natural conception [17] however, many studies show that these risks are low and further reduced when surgery is performed laparoscopically [18]. The fear of potential effects of pregnancy and delivery on the pouch or passing on a genetic mutation in FAP and increased age increases infertility rates post RPC [19]. Women over the age of 35 or those with recognised fertility problems, such as history of pelvic surgery, should consult their GP after 6 months of unprotected sex without conception [20].

Sperm banking is not routinely recommended as RPC does not impede the production of sperm however distribution may be compromised in the presence of erectile dysfunction, retrograde or dry ejaculation [21]. If these conditions persist, patients may be referred to an infertility specialist to have sperm retrieval for storage or insemination at a later date. However, if a patient requires pelvic radiotherapy, sperm banking and egg harvesting must be discussed as the production and quality of sperm and eggs may be affected. NICE guidelines recommend women under 40 years of age to have unprotected intercourse for 2 years before being considered for in vitro fertilization (IVF) [22].

## 11.5 Contraception

It is equally important to discuss contraception and family planning, as many young patients may not be in a position to start a family immediately post RPC. Contraceptive pills are mainly absorbed within the duodenum, therefore patients with a pouch will usually absorb drugs effectively [12] however care must be taken if patients have prolonged episodes of diarrhoea and vomiting as this may reduce the efficacy of medication. There is a lack of scientific evidence supporting the ability of commonly prescribed antibiotics to reduce the effectiveness of oral contraceptives (with the exception of rifampin and rifabutin), however patients on long-term or combination antibiotic therapy may be prone to episodes of diarrhoea which can reduce absorption of oral contraception [23]. Other forms of acceptable contraception are condoms, diaphragms, implants and 3 monthly depot injections. The intrauterine device (IUD) or coil has been used following RPC though discussions with a family planning specialist is advised and should not be recommended in nulliparous women. Long term contraception methods such as vasectomy or sterilisation may be suitable alternatives. Sterilisation via an abdominal or vaginal approach warrants a discussion with a colorectal surgeon.

## 11.6 Pregnancy and Delivery

During pregnancy, many women experience deteriorating continence and increased pouch frequency caused by the mechanical and hormonal effects of pregnancy, particularly in the third trimester [11]. It is important for the PNP to reassure and support these patients as symptoms usually normalise promptly post-partum [10]. Changes to the inflammatory system, dietary requirements, fluid balance and lifestyle in pregnancy, potentially have an adverse effect on pouch function. The use of anti-diarrhoeal medication such as *Loperamide Hydrochloride* is not usually recommended in pregnancy therefore barrier creams and pads may be required to maintain perianal comfort. *Co-amoxiclav* may be used for suitable pregnant patients with increased frequency secondary to pouchitis [24].

There still remains controversy on the optimal method of delivery following RPC. Women are advised to opt for a caesarean section as a traumatic vaginal delivery can result in occult sphincter damage which may impede future pouch function [8]. A well-managed vaginal delivery is not impossible for women who wish to experience a natural birth. Patients should be encouraged to discuss the preferred mode of delivery with their obstetrician and surgeon so appropriate plans can be put in place [25].

## 11.7 Post-operative Care

Given the complexity of RPC and long-term post-operative care required, patients benefit by being treated in an experienced networked unit [26, 27]. RPC requires two or three surgical hospital admissions, where direct advice, supervision and support is vital for patient safety and satisfaction.

Many of the early complications post RPC are managed successfully in the acute hospital setting by a multidisciplinary approach in which the PNP has roles such as managing high output ileostomy, peri-stomal complications or initial stoma or pouch-anal stenosis requiring dilation or catheterisation.

Familiarity, trust and understanding between the PNP and the patient gained through extensive pre-operative assessment and routine post-operative support, re-enforces the patient's knowledge and prepares them to manage effectively through the multiple operative phases of RPC. This affiliation places the PNP in the best position to offer long-term lifestyle advice in order to achieve the best results possible from the pouch.

## 11.8 Stoma Care

Stoma care is commonly the patient's main apprehension once committed to RPC. An ileostomy is life changing and adaptation may be challenging despite the ileostomy being a temporary fixture. However some patients perceive an ileostomy as relief to the debilitating symptoms of their disease and a step towards improving quality of life. Adaptation to the ileostomy is not without struggle, as stoma care can be a distressing and unpleasant experience, especially in the first few weeks post-operatively. Few patients may not experience an ileostomy due to body habitus, a shortened mesentery or insufficient length of ileum intra-operatively or if they were intentionally selected for one stage or modified two stage RPC. Techniques which avoid an ileostomy remain controversial due to the associated risks involved [28].

Following RPC with loop ileostomy, the patient is generally in an improved state both physically and mentally in contrast to their initial colectomy with an end ileostomy. They are also better prepared in regards to stoma care and general recovery. Stoma care may become more challenging with a loop ileostomy and it is common for patients to require a high output or convex appliance, accessory stoma products and re-education on diet and fluid balance to prevent dehydration. Patients are reassured that blood or mucous loss and the sensation to evacuate the newly formed pouch is not uncommon.

Although RPC is performed to avoid a permanent ileostomy, the role of the PNP is to ensure the patient's experience of living with the ileostomy is made as positive as possible. In the unfortunate circumstance of pouch failure, patients anecdotally tend to accept a permanent ileostomy easier if they were well supported, fully informed and not exposed to multiple traumatic experiences when living with a stoma.

## 11.9 Ileostomy Closure

The ileostomy will be closed approximately 3 months post RPC when the pouch anal anastomosis is confirmed by pouchogram to be intact. This final operation is minor in comparison to previous surgery but possibly the most challenging for the patient. Stoma closure marks the end of the patients' medical support network, as they no longer have a disease process or an ileostomy. However for the experienced PNP, another journey takes form with the patient and their new pouch. Adaptive changes within the pouch such as bacterial colonisation [29] and reinstating of autonomic fibres, may take up to 12 months to stabilise pouch performance. Patience, support and reassurance from the PNP is vital in order for the patient to gain confidence in pouch function.

The PNP will reinstate the following at stoma closure:

- Anal skin care advice and provide a selection of barrier creams or wipes
- Urge resistance techniques to manage pouch frequency
- Techniques to defer defecation
- Toileting positions to assist in evacuation of the pouch
- Anti-motility medication usage, titrated to bowel function
- Diet and fluid management
- Returning to work and general lifestyle advice
- Structured nurse-led follow up and support should complications arise

## 11.10 Perianal Skin Care

Initially following ileostomy closure it is expected that the pouch frequency will be erratic and leakage and seepage may occur especially at night. The effluent is rich in digestive enzymes that can easily break down healthy perianal skin. Pruritus ani is a frequent complaint, occurring when faecal effluent makes contact with the anal canal and can be exacerbated with frequent wiping [30]. It is important to educate patients on good anal hygiene and skin care immediately after ileostomy closure (Fig. 11.1). If anal pain is extreme or persistent, anal fissures, abscess formation or fistula-in-ano should be excluded.

## 11.11 Dietary Advice

The availability of vast, multi-cultural diets combined with fast paced, erratic lifestyles of some pouch patients can make choosing food increasingly difficult. Initially after stoma closure patients are advised to consume a light, low residue diet, avoiding high fibre, raw or uncooked fruit and vegetables for 3–4 weeks. Starchy carbohydrates such as white varieties of bread, pasta, rice and potatoes

**Clean:**

- Use soft tissue and/or wet wipes
- Refrain from excess wiping as this can exacerbate matters
- If perineum particularly sore wash area directly with shower head or sit in a shallow warm bath
- Ensure anal area is completely clean from residual cream and faecal matter
- Refrain from using wipes with scents or disinfectant as these can irritate broken skin

**Dry:**

- Dab dry with soft wipe or tissue
- Ensure anal area is clean and dry before next step

**Wear:**

- Apply small amount of suitable barrier cream or barrier film
- Apply small amount of barrier cream inside the anal canal
- Wear loose fitting cotton underwear

**Fig. 11.1** Anal skin care advice

(without skins) should be included in every meal. These adjustments are required initially to prevent bowel obstruction, excessive odour, abdominal bloating and high or unpredictable output from the pouch. The majority of established pouch patients report the ability to eat a well-balanced, varied diet successfully, which includes moderate consumption of alcohol. Most patients will not feel comfortable to pass flatus without sitting on the toilet for fear of involuntary soiling, therefore taking note of the foods which adversely affect pouch function is highly important, though very individual.

Some foods or drinks may consistently cause concern and should be avoided or ingested sparingly. Spicy foods, nuts, citrus or dried fruits, citrus juice, red wine, popcorn and coconut are notorious for disrupting pouch function and worth noting as may be the contributing factor of a bowel obstruction. Vegans and vegetarians are no more likely to have difficulties choosing suitable foods because their bowel is well adapted to the particular dietary choices prior to RPC.

## 11.12 Nurse-Led Clinics

The pivotal nurse-led pouch clinic was established at St. Mark's Hospital in the late 1990's not only to offer consistent long-term care to patients following RPC but to support and potentially reduce the workload of the surgical teams. In addition to the traditional roles of ileostomy siting and stoma care, the PNP is now well established within the field of gastroenterology with extensions of the role involving independent diagnosis, advanced counselling skills, non-medical prescribing, physical assessment, such as digital examination and rigid pouchoscopy [31, 32]. Data collected from these clinics has been used to structure the follow up requirements of pouch patients, design national protocols and to promote evidence based, best practice guidelines, whilst shaping the future of nurse-led services. Nurse-led care has shown improvements in time management, patient experience, access to care, effectiveness of consultations and reduced patient waiting times [33].

## 11.13 Long Term Nurse-Led Follow Up

The PNP's main influence on patient experience appears to be in managing the patient immediately post ileostomy reversal, with a newly functioning ileoanal pouch and continuing regular assessment and timely interventions as required in an outpatient setting. In high volume institutions where staffing levels and training permits, the PNP role is exclusive to patients considering or undergoing RPC, or those who have unfortunately reverted to a permanent ileostomy following pouch failure.

In other hospitals, the PNP role is incorporated within the stoma care nursing model however most stoma nurses are not responsible for the ongoing assessment of pouch patients and do not necessarily have the experience of dealing with the complexities arising from RPC.

Changes within healthcare delivery modes, such as the advent of virtual clinics and telephone/email interventions, allow suitable pouch patients to be monitored or reviewed remotely by the PNP. Cases which require physical assessment in order to obtain a correct diagnosis are an obvious limitation to these assessment methods.

Structured follow-up for pouch patients on the background of FAP is evident but there remains controversy on the ideal duration or method of follow-up for patients with a pouch on the background of UC. Follow-up varies between surgical or medical care pending upon institution and presenting complication type. Ideally, complex patients should be managed by a multi-disciplinary approach involving surgical, medical and nursing input.

For patients with a background of UC, a 6 week nurse-led PNP clinic appointment is made following stoma closure with patients routinely discharged from Consultant care. Nurse-led interventions are then arranged at 3, 6 and 12 months. Consultations are based on validated quality of life questionnaires and assessed on an individual basis. Patients are discharged from routine PNP care at 12 months unless they presented with dysplasia, rectal carcinoma or primary sclerosing cholangitis at colectomy or present with refractory pouchitis. Lifelong support should be readily available for all pouch patients in the form of outpatient clinics, email and telephone advice lines.

## 11.14 Medication Advice

The advent of non-medical prescribing has broken down boundaries within healthcare and extended the prescribing rights of specialist nurses allowing them to provide a seamless service to ileoanal pouch patients, with the aim of improving patient experience and overall quality of life [33, 34].

In line with national guidelines surrounding advance practice and nurse-led clinics, the pouch nurse can order diagnostic investigations and prescribe necessary preparatory medication for pouchoscopy, independently follow-up the outcomes of such investigations, discharge or monitor patients with specific long-term conditions, such as pouchitis and prescribe and alter treatment medication in line with the Nursing and Midwifery (NMC) prescribing guidelines [35], national and local protocols.

Most patients with a protracted history of UC report a desire to reduce or eliminate the use of medication post RPC following years of disease treatment requiring polypharmacy or complex mediation regimes. However, there are some inherent benefits of medication use with an ileoanal pouch such as improved faecal consistency and therefore better evacuation or in the management of recurrent inflammation or post-operative sepsis. Typically the drugs of choice are usually easy to administer, the medication course brief and adverse effects limited in the long term. Medication may be in form of tablets, an elixir or be administered directly into the pouch via an enema or suppository.

Self-diagnosis and self-medication appears to be prominent with ileoanal pouch patients in order for them to manage bowel frequency and demanding lifestyle routines, consistent with modern day living, yet this phenomenon is severely under reported in the literature. The paucity of information is likely due to unrecognised or unreported self-mediation practices and the increased use of alternate therapies, off label and unlicensed medications prescribed for pouch patients. However, there may be a correlation between self-medication practices and the advice and support patients receive post-operation. Emerging data states that institutional volume has a significant association to ileoanal pouch failure [26], suggesting that lack of specialist knowledge in the field of ileoanal pouch surgery could lead to patients being managed incorrectly and therefore resorting to inappropriate self-care and medication habits.

Appropriate self-medication has been linked to several benefits such as reduced anxiety for the patient, increased access to mediation, improvements in self-care, better use of health care resources and clinicians' time and skills. However irresponsible self-medication, incorrect self-diagnosis, delays in seeking medical advice, incorrect drug dose, duration or administration, can lead to adverse side effects, ineffective treatment and dependence or resistance to certain medication [36]. The PNP is therefore in an ideal position to coordinate long-term lifestyle and medication requirements to ensure best practice guidelines are observed.

## 11.15 Nurse-Led Complication Diagnosis, Treatment and Management

A large proportion of patient queries surround changes to normal pouch routine, mediation advice, complication diagnosis and management techniques. The main presenting complaints discussed with the PNP are:

### *11.15.1 Increased Frequency and Urgency*

Commonly patients have misconceptions surrounding pouch function therefore can be unduly concerned with changes in pouch frequency or urgency. In most cases evacuation frequency can be controlled with the consistent use of anti-motility drugs, which most patients are accustomed to preceding ileostomy reversal. *Lomatil* was the original anti-motility medication used in clinical trials to prolong intestinal transit and reduce bowel frequency following stoma closure after RPC [37], however it has since been replaced by *Loperamide Hydrochloride* (Immodium® or Norimode®). Loperamide can be acquired either over the counter or on prescription. It is especially useful in patients with a pouch as it improves anal sphincter function which maintains continence and may also assist to reduce the sensations associated with urgency [38]. Loperamide has only one reported drug interaction and most patients do not report the predictable side effects such as dizziness, flatulence or nausea, making the drug reaction profile low [24].

Some pouch patients report Loperamide causing evacuation difficulties at low doses therefore care must be taken to increase the dose slowly whilst monitoring the effectiveness. Doses range from 2 to 16 mg daily with an unlicensed indication of up to 32 mg daily, however select patients may be prescribed significantly higher doses. It is paramount that the patient is included in administration decisions to improve concordance and adherence to medication regimes, as most patients neglect to take Loperamide 30–40 min before meals which offers better efficacy. On the rare occasion that Loperamide capsules are passed through the ileoanal pouch, the capsules can be opened or tablets crushed and sprinkled onto food [39]. Loperamide elixir may be used however the volume required is usually high with increased cost implications. Taking drugs multiple times a day and over a protracted period of time has its own challenges such as reduced compliance and therefore some patients benefit from larger doses less frequently [40].

Patients are advised to allow the ileoanal pouch to become accustomed to its new role before introducing Loperamide and therefore most patients are not routinely prescribed anti-motility drugs immediately post ileostomy closure. Therefore it is recommended that the optimal time to commence Loperamide is discussed on an individual basis and reviewed according to lifestyle and daily frequency.

Opioid drugs such as *Codeine Phosphate* can be prescribed to improve faecal consistency after ileostomy closure. In concentrated, regular doses Codeine based analgesia is known to be addictive, sedative and documented as the cause of fat malabsorption [41, 42]. However the combined use of Loperamide and low dose Codeine Phosphate appears to be effective in some pouch patients. *Codeine* combined with *Paracetamol* can be effective in patients with abdominal pain and pouch frequency.

*Ispaghula Husk* (Fybogel™, Psyllium Husk™) is a bulk-forming laxative that increases faecal mass and may be useful in reducing ileoanal pouch frequency however the effect may take a couple of days to become apparent. Some patients find no obvious benefit from such preparations and others may experience excess flatus, bloating and abdominal cramping and therefore bulk-forming laxatives are not be suitable for all pouch patients.

*Amitriptyline* is an anti-depressant however in very low doses it is helpful in reducing the pouch frequency if this is caused by an 'over sensitive' pouch. Amitriptyline is also used to help with nerve pain especially in the anus, in the presence of tenesmus [43] or in irritable pouch syndrome.

### *11.15.2 Leakage and Seepage*

Minor incontinence from the pouch can be a frustrating adaptation for some patients after ileostomy reversal usually occurring at night, during exercise or mobilising considerable distances. The PNP will encourage pelvic floor exercises, diet and medication changes to encourage the effluent to remain in the pouch. Reassurance is vital in the early days to remind patients that the sphincter muscles will take time to adapt to evacuation after a period of redundancy. Patients will be instructed to use barrier creams and wipes to prevent a sore perineum. The use of thin sanitary wear or folded tissue between the buttocks can be effective, utilizing larger pads as required. Men may benefit using triangle shaped pads as they are more comfortable. Leakage that continues to cause discomfort should be investigated and referred for anal physiology and manometry to detect any defects within the anal canal or biofeedback to enhance evacuation techniques and pouch compliance.

### *11.15.3 Pouchitis*

Pouchitis is the most commonly diagnosed complication in the literature [44] and patients are managed based on the protocol for pouch dysfunction and pouchitis [45] which is illustrated within chapter 9 on pouchitis. It is paramount to take a full medical history and if possible perform a flexible pouchoscopy with biopsy to ascertain the possible cause of dysfunction and to avoid misdiagnosis. Increased frequency and urgency may be associated with pouchitis but this is not always the case, as unresolved sepsis in or around the pouch, may present with similar symptoms.

Patients need to be conscious of their normal frequency as this may differ considerably from the frequency quoted in the literature. Unrelenting pouchitis or antibiotic resistant pouchitis is associated with a reduced quality of life [46] and may result in pouch failure therefore early detection and management of pouchitis is essential.

Consistent PNP review ensures patients are not lost to follow-up and the appropriate clinical investigations or complex medical regimes are maintained. Patients on long-term antibiotics are monitored in outpatient or telephone clinics reducing consultant or GP involvement. The PNP can also triage suitable patients onto current drug trials, offer assistance to patients for the duration of the trial, as well as assisting with vital data collection.

### 11.15.4 Cuffitis

Inflammation of the columnar cuff can be difficult to treat and may require long term use (6 weeks) of *Mesalazine suppositories* [47] (also known as Asacol®, Pentasa® or Salofalk®), *Prednisolone suppositories* or Predfoam® *enemas.* These can be self-administered into the pouch with remote guidance from the PNP. Suppositories tend to work better as they remain in the pouch longer than an enema and patients are advised to administer medication at a time when evacuation is reduced, for example at night.

### 11.15.5 Abdominal, Anal or Pelvic Pain

Most patients report intermittent abdominal and anal pain following ileostomy closure. This is usually short lived and resolved with variations in diet and lifestyle or with the use of simple analgesia. Ongoing pelvic pain warrants further investigation such as radiological investigations or MRI to exclude pelvic sepsis, anastomotic leak or fistula formation.

Analgesics such as *Paracetamol and Codeine Phosphate* may be effective for pain relief with Codeine having the benefit of thickening the stool. However Codeine can increase abdominal discomfort with excess use may even compromise evacuation. *Hyoscine butylbromide* (Buscopan®) can be used to help with bowel spasms or windy and cramping pain. *Peppermint derivatives* in water, oil and capsules can calm abdominal pain associated with bloating.

*Non-steroidal anti-inflammatory drugs (NSAIDS)* should be avoided as they can cause macroscopic injury to the small intestine resulting in ulceration of the pouch and ineffective mucosal healing [48]. NSAID induced pouchitis is documented in the literature as a secondary identifiable/triggering factor of pouchitis in patients with regular use of this medication [49].

### 11.15.6 Bowel Obstruction

Dietary related bowel obstructions are common and usually resolve by patients discontinuing diet, increasing fluid intake and instructing techniques such as abdominal massage, relaxation techniques, sitting in a warm bath or gentle exercise to spontaneously resolve the blockage. If patients are nauseated an anti-emetic drug may be advised in combination with non-constipating, analgesic medication.

Unremitting obstructions due to luminal strictures or bowel rotation/twisting causing vomiting and reduced or ceased bowel movements warrants immediate medical intervention. In this instance the first line advice is intravenous analgesia and fluid, with radiological investigation. Patients may benefit from nasal gastric tube insertion and remaining nil by mouth until the obstruction is resolved. Surgery is not normally required and should not be suggested as first line treatment.

### 11.15.7 Dehydration

Dehydration occurs periodically with most pouch patients as they are fairly young, physically active and not always observant to the early signs of dehydration. Patients are advised to drink one and a half to two litres of water per day but to also add approximately one teaspoon of salt to their diet as routine. Avoiding excessive amounts of caffeine or cola is useful as this may act as a diuretic. If patients undergo strenuous exercise, participate in sport or experience increased pouch frequency, vomiting or diarrhoea, rehydration fluids are also advised.

### 11.15.8 Rehydration Fluids

*Dioralyte®* is a standard rehydration drink however patients with an ileoanal pouch are recommended to use concentrated, double strength Dioralyte® (10 sachets in 1 litre of water). Concentrated Dioralyte® has a high dose of potassium and must be used with caution in long term use therefore blood serology should be requested if concerned. *St. Mark's Hospital Electrolyte Mix* is an alternative rehydration drink with easily acquired powdered components (Fig. 11.2). The solution expires after 24 h.

*Isotonic drinks* such as Lucozade™, PowerAde™, Gatorade™ replace fluid and some electrolytes and are convenient for immediate use. The sport varieties are

**St. Mark's Hospital Electrolyte Mix**

This recipe uses the measurements in 5ml teaspoons:

- Six level teaspoons of Glucose powder (20g)
- One level teaspoon of Sodium Chloride, which is table salt (3.5g)
- Half a heaped teaspoon of Sodium Bicarbonate, also called Bicarbonate of Soda (2.5g)

Add all the ingredients into ONE litre of water

Stir the contents until dissolved

Chill in the refrigerator, as it is more palatable to drink

Do not add ice as this will dilute the solution but a splash of cordial may improve the taste.

The solution will last for 24 hours.

All of the ingredients for St. Mark's Hospital Electrolyte Mix can be found in a supermarket or chemist and will not require a prescription.

**Fig. 11.2** St. Mark's Hospital electrolyte mix recipe

advised, which are non-carbonated and may contain less sugar. However isotonic drinks do not contain enough electrolytes for long term use.

### *11.15.9 Incomplete Evacuation*

In order to assist evacuation patients are advised to manipulate their position on the toilet. Some patients find that they will need to stand up and sit back down again, massage their abdomen and try different positions in order to achieve a feeling of complete evacuation. It is important to advise patients not to strain. If positioning does not help evacuation it may be necessary to instruct the patient to use a Medena catheter. Medena catherterisation has shown clinical benefits to patients with functional or mechanical problems resulting in incomplete evacuation or difficulties initiating evacuation [31]. Some patients with a retained rectal remnant, angulation of

**Patient Instructions on Medena Catheterisation**

**Equipment: Medena catheter, lubricating gel, bladder syringe and tepid tap water**

- Fill the syringe with tepid tap water.
- Lubricate the end of the Medena catheter and eyelets with lubricating gel and also the anal area.
- Hold the catheter between the thumb and forefinger, approximately 6-10 cm from the eyelets.
- Depending on which is more comfortable, insert the catheter into the anus whilst stooping or sitting on the toilet. Stop when your fingers reach the buttocks.
- Ensure the other end of the Medena catheter is aimed towards the toilet bowl.
- When the Medena catheter is in the correct position flatus or faecal fluid will drain.

You can help ensure the pouch is empty by wiggling your hips, gently massaging the abdomen or coughing. It may be useful to stand up and then sit down again. If the stool is not draining, the catheter may need a flush. Attach the bladder syringe to the end of the catheter and gently flush with 20-30mls of water. To remove, pull downwards whilst gently rolling between your fingers. The Medena catheter is re-usable so can be washed in soapy water and then dried. You may need to use a catheter for every bowel motion or as advised by your pouch nurse.

**Fig. 11.3** Patient instructions on how to use a medena catheter

the pouch anal anastomosis or an 'S' shaped configuration pouch also benefit from using a Medena. Imaging such as a defaecating pouchogram may support the use of a Medena catheter however this is not always clinically indicative [50]. The PNP will provide written and verbal instructions on how to use the Medena and monitor patient progress (Fig. 11.3). Medena catheters are available on prescription described as 'ileostomy catheters' (Fig. 11.4).

### *11.15.10 Pouch Anal Anastomotic Stricture*

Misdiagnosis of pouch anal anastomotic stricture is common, as patients may present with a multitude of symptoms such as increased or reduced pouch frequency, urgency, erratic pouch function, incomplete evacuation and occasionally bleeding. The use of a Hegar dilator may be helpful after digital examination and confirmation of the stricture. Some patients may initially need surgical dilation of the pouch anal anastomosis prior to the long term use of a Hegar dilator to ensure the anastomosis remains patent.

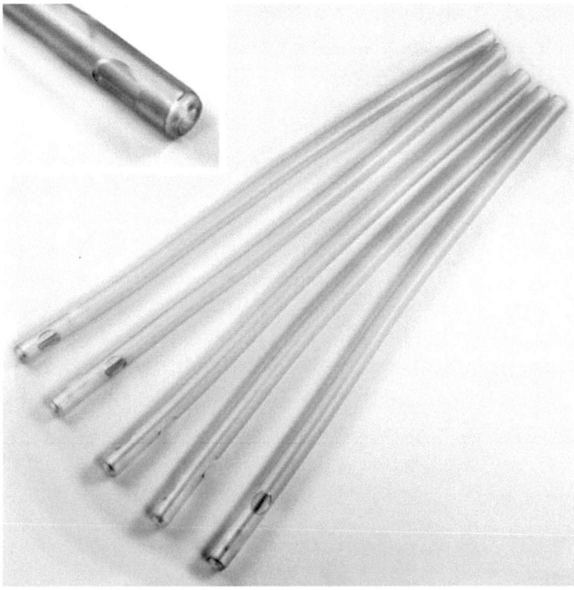

**Fig. 11.4** Medena catheter

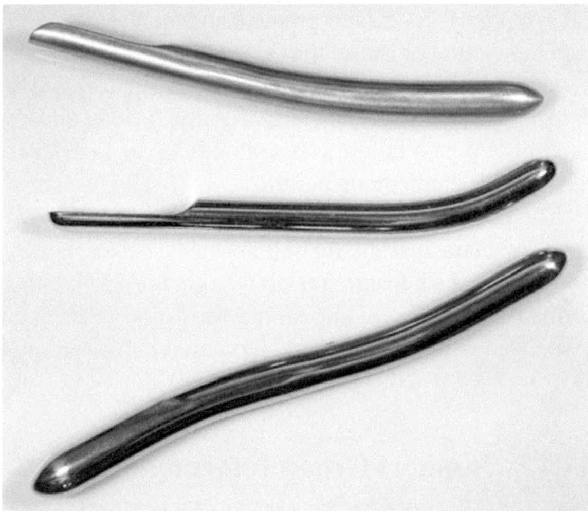

**Fig. 11.5** Hegar dilators

Hegar dilators are available in various sizes and as single or doubled ended dilators (Fig. 11.5). The most commonly prescribed sizes range from 15 to 18 mm. If Hegar dilators are not available on prescription, they can be purchased for under £10 online. The PNP will advise the patient to lubricate the Hegar dilator and observe them as they gently insert the dilator into the anus and through the pouch anal anastomosis. Frequency of use depends on the history of the patient and their lifestyle. Initially most patients are advised to use the Hegar daily, however this time can be extended as long as the patient is comfortable that the anastomotic stricture has not reoccurred. Ideally patients with a history of anastomotic strictures are advised to use the dilator at least weekly for as long as they have the pouch.

### *11.15.11 Anal Fissure*

Anal fissure can present at any time but early diagnosis should made with patients who rely on regular Medena catheterisation or dilation of the pouch as fissures can become cyclical and treatment difficult. The use of *Diltiazem 2% cream* or *Glyceryl Trinitrate 0.4% ointment should* be applied directly to the affected area. This will increase blood flow to the anus and assist healing.

## 11.16 Pouch Failure

Pouch failure presents as a regression towards UC, with not only debilitating physical symptoms, but disappointment and mental anguish for the patient. The treatment is to defunction or excise the ileoanal pouch and form a permanent ileostomy. Some patients live with a poor quality of life solely to avoid the physical and social stigma associated with a permanent ileostomy. A deep understanding of the patient's perception of pouch failure is essential in order to offer realistic support and management in this challenging period.

The risk of pouch failure is approximately 9% at 5 years and 12% at 10 years with the main reasons for failure being pelvic sepsis, chronic antibiotic resistant pouchitis and idiopathic pouch dysfunction [51]. Other factors such as low annual hospital volume, avoiding stoma formation at RPC and female gender were also associated with a significantly increased risk of failure [52].

## 11.17 Support Group Information

The PNP is not always the best person to explain the lived experience following surgery. Patients report benefits to speaking with other people who have undergone RPC. Access to medical information, psychological support, personal blogs and visual aids via social media and the internet are widely utilised [53]. Most charities and support organisations have websites, while some provide interactive chat rooms or advice lines. For patients who prefer face to face meetings these can also be arranged directly via the organisation or through the PNP. Patients who are well informed, prepared and supported through their pouch surgery usually have better outcomes and can manage complications more effectively.

St. Mark's Hospital is the largest centre for ileoanal pouches in the UK and the only centre with dedicated pouch nurses.

Telephone advice line 0208 235 4126

Email: lnwh-tr.internalpouchcare@nhs.net

Website: www.stmarkshospital.org.uk

Ileostomy and Internal Pouch Support Group (IA). The IA is a UK registered charity whose primary aim is to help people who have to undergo surgery and are now living with an ileostomy or an ileo-anal pouch, their families, friends and carers.

Telephone: 0800 0184 724

Email: info@iasupport.org

Website: www.iasupport.org

The Red Lion Group is a UK pouch support charity for people who have or are considering having, an ileo-anal pouch. The pouch support group was founded in 1994 by a group of patients and staff at St. Mark's Hospital in London and gained charitable status in 1997. The Group provides a forum for patients and their friends and family to share best practice, top tips and information on pouch-related matters.

Email: liaison@redliongroup.org

Website: www.redliongroup.org

## References


1. Shen B. Problems after restorative proctocolectomy: assessment and therapy. Curr Opin Gastroenterol. 2016;32(1):49–54.
2. Salehimarzijarni B, Jalay N, Dadvar Z, et al. Long term quality of life after ileal anal restorative proctocolectomy for ulcerative colitis. Indian J Gastroenterol. 2012;31(1):49–53.
3. Scoglio D, Ahmed Ali U, Fichera A. Surgical treatment of ulcerative colitis: Ileorectal vs ileal pouch-anal anastomosis. World J Gastroenterol. 2014;20(37):13211–8.
4. Misra R, Askari A, Faiz O, et al. Colectomy rates for ulcerative colitis differ between ethnic groups: results from a 15-year Nationwide cohort study. Can J Gastroenterol Hepatol. 2016; https://doi.org/10.1155/2016/8723949.
5. Perry-Woodford Z. Quality of life following ileoanal pouch failure. Br J Nurs. 2014;22(Suppl. 16):S23–8.
6. Carmon E, Keidar A. The correlation between quality of life and functional outcome in ulcerative colitis patients after proctocolectomy ileal pouch anal anastomosis. Color Dis. 2003;5(3):228–32.
7. Forsmo H, Pfeffer F, Rasdal A, et al. Pre- and postoperative stoma education and guidance with an enhanced recovery after surgery (ERAS) programme reduces length of hospital stay in colorectal surgery. Int J Surg. 2016;36:121–6.
8. Nicholls J, Williams J. The ileo anal pouch in Burch J. (2008) The essentials of pouch care nursing. London: Whurr Publishers; 2002.
9. Sunde M, Oresland T, Faerden T. Correlation between pouch function and sexual function in patients with IPAA. Scand J Gastroenterol. 2016;51(3):295–303.
10. Delaini G, Scaglia M, Colucci G, et al. The ileoanal pouch procedure in the long–term perspective: a critical review. Tech Coloproctol. 2005;9(3):187–92.
11. Cornish J, Tan E, Teare J, et al. The effect of restorative proctocolectomy on sexual function, urinary function, fertility, pregnancy and delivery: a systematic review. Dis Colon Rectum. 2007;50(8):1128–38.
12. Williams J. The essentials of pouch care nursing. London: Whurr Publishers Ltd; 2002.
13. Vella M, Masood M, Hendry W, et al. Surgery for ulcerative colitis. R Coll Surg Edinburgh Ireland. 2007;5(6):356–62.
14. Kjaer M, Laursen S, Qvist N, et al. Sexual function and body image are similar after laparoscopy-assisted and open ileal pouch-anal anastomosis. World J Surg. 2014;38(9):2460–5.
15. Borwell B (1997) Ileoanal pouch surgery and its after care in Williams J. The essentials of pouch care nursing. London: Whurr Publishers; 2002.
16. Hor T, Lefevre J, Shields C, et al. Female sexual function and fertility after ileal pouch-anal anastomosis. Int J Colorectal Dis. 2016;31(3):593–601.
17. Valente M, Hull T. Fertility and delivery after IPAA. Società Italiana di Chirurgia Colo Rettale. 2014;41:355–45.
18. Konishi T, Ishida H, Ueno H, et al. Feasibility of laparoscopic total proctocolectomy with ileal pouch–anal anastomosis and total colectomy with ileorectal anastomosis for familial adenomatous polyposis: results of a nationwide multicenter study. Int J Clin Oncol. 2016;21:953–61.
19. Olsen K, Juul S, Bulows S, et al. Female fecundity before and after operation for familial adenomatous polyposis. Br J Surg. 2003;90:227–31.
20. NHS choices. Fertility requirements before seeking advice. Available from http://www.nhs.uk/conditions/infertility/pages/introduction.aspx
21. Burch J. Stoma care. Chichester: Wiley; 2008.
22. NICE guidelines for fertility problem: assessment and treatment. Clinical guideline (CG156) 2013. Updated Sep 2017. Available from https://www.nice.org.uk/guidance/cg156/chapter/Recommendations#access-criteria-for-ivf
23. De Rossi D, Hersh E. Antibiotics and oral contraceptives. Dent Clin N Am. 2002;46(4):653–64.
24. Joint Formulary Committee. British National Formulary. 70th ed. London: BMJ Group and Pharmaceutical Press; 2016.

25. Øresland T, Bemelman A, Spinelli A, et al. ECCO guidelines/consensus paper, European evidence based consensus on surgery for ulcerative colitis. J Crohns Colitis. 2014;9:4–25.
26. Burns E, Bottle A, Aylin P, et al. Volume analysis of outcome following restorative proctocolectomy. Br J Surg. 2011;98(3):408–17.
27. Association of Coloproctology of Great Britain and Ireland (ACPGBI) Ileoanal pouch report (cited 2017 Oct 6) available from https://www.acpgbi.org.uk/resources/
28. Sofo L, Caprino P, Franco Sacchetti F, et al. Restorative proctocolectomy with ileal pouch-anal anastomosis for ulcerative colitis: a narrative review. World J Gastrointest Surg. 2016;8(8):556–63.
29. Falk A, Olsson C, Ahrné S, et al. Ileal pelvic pouch microbiota from two former ulcerative colitis patients, analysed by DNA-based methods, were unstable over time and showed the presence of Clostridium perfringens. Scand J Gastroenterol. 2007;42(8):973–85.
30. Mason I. Continence care for patients with inflammatory bowel disease. Nurs Stand. 2007;22(8):43–6.
31. Perry-Woodford Z, McLaughlin S. Recommended follow-up for ileo-anal pouch patient. Br J Nurs. 2008;17(4):220–4.
32. Perrin A. Development of a nurse-led ileo-anal pouch clinic. Br J Nurs. 2005;14(16):S21–4.
33. Randall S, Crawford T, Currie J, et al. Impact of community based nurse-led clinics on patient outcomes, patient satisfaction, patient access and cost effectiveness: a systematic review. J Nurs Stud. 2017;73:24–33.
34. Carey N, Stenner K. Does non-medical prescribing make a difference to patients? Nurs Times. 2011;107(26):14–6.
35. Standards of proficiency for nurse and midwife prescribers, nursing and midwifery council (NMC 2006). Available at https://www.nmc.org.uk/standards/additional-standards/standards-of-proficiency-for-nurse-and-midwife-prescribers/
36. Ruiz M. Risks of self-medication practices. Curr Drug Saf. 2010;5(4):315–23.
37. Pemberton J, Kelly K, Beart R, et al. Ileal pouch-anal anastomosis for chronic ulcerative colitis: long-term results. Ann Surg. 1987;206:504–13.
38. Hallgren T, Fasth S, Delbro D, et al. Loperamide improves anal sphincter function and continence after restorative proctocolectomy. Dig Dis. 1994;39(12):2612–8.
39. Nightingale J, Woodward J. Guidelines for management of patients with a short bowel. Gut. 2006;55(Suppl. 4):iv1–iv12.
40. Tungaraza T, Talapan-Manikoth P, Jenkins R. Curse of the ghost pills: the role of oral controlled-release formulations in the passage of empty intact shells in faeces. Two case reports and a literature review relevant to psychiatry. Ther Adv Drug Saf. 4(2):63–71.
41. Ruppin H. Review: loperamide--a potent antidiarrhoeal drug with actions along the alimentary tract. Aliment Pharmacol Ther. 1987;1(3):179–90.
42. Mackowski A, Chen H, Levitt M. Successful management of chronic high-output ileostomy with high dose Loperamide. Br Med J case report. Published online:28 March 2015. https://doi.org/10.1136/bcr-2015-209411.
43. Livovsky D, Adler S, Adar T, et al. Tricyclic antidepressants for the treatment of tenesmus associated with rectal prolapse. Colorectal Dis. 2015;17(12):1094–9.
44. Helavirta I, Huhtala H, Hyöty MP, et al. Restorative proctocolectomy for ulcerative colitis 1985–2009. Scand J Surg. 2016;105(2):73–7.
45. Segal J, Ding N, Worley G, et al. Systematic review with meta-analysis: the management of the chronic refractory pouchitis with an evidenced based treatment algorithm. Aliment Pharmacol Ther. 2016; n/a-n/a. https://doi.org/10.1111/apt.13905.
46. McLaughlin S, Clark S, Tekkis P, et al. An open study of maintenance antibiotic therapy for chronic antibiotic-dependent pouchitis:efficacy, complications and outcome. Colorectal Dis. 2011;13(4):438–44.
47. Shen B, Lashner B, Bennet M, et al. Treatment of rectal cuff inflammation (cuffitis) in patients with ulcerative colitis following restorative proctocolectomy with ileal pouch anal anastomosis. Am J Gastroenterol. 2004;99:1527–31.

48. Maiden L, Thjodleifsson B, Theodors A, et al. A quantitative analysis of NSAID-induced small bowel pathology by capsule enteroscopy. Gastroenterology. 2005;128(5):1172–8.
49. Navaneethan U, Shen B. Secondary pouchitis: those with identifiable etiopathogenetic or triggering factors. Am J Gastroenterol. 2010;105:51–64.
50. Stellingwerf M, Maeda Y, Patel U, et al. The role of the defaecating pouchogram in the assessment of evacuation difficulty after restorative proctocolectomy and pouch anal anastomosis. Colorectal Dis. 2016;18:0292–300.
51. Tulchinsky H, Hawley P, Subba Rao K, et al. Long-term failure after restorative proctocolectomy for ulcerative colitis. Ann Surg. 2003;238(2):229–34.
52. Mark-Christensen A, Erichsen R, Brandsborg S, et al. Pouch failures following ileal pouch-anal anastomosis for ulcerative colitis. Color Dis. Accepted Author Manuscript. https://doi.org/10.1111/codi.13802.
53. Perry-Woodford Z, Segal J, Clark S, et al. Assessing online information sources on ileal pouch-anal anastomosis. Gastrointest Nurs. 2017;15(1):2.

# Chapter 12
# Optimising Pouch Function Using Biofeedback

**Brigitte Collins and Elissa Bradshaw**

**Abstract** Biofeedback therapy is an effective treatment for bowel dysfunction. The service at the Sir Alan Parks Physiology and Neuromodulation Unit has been successful in providing biofeedback therapy for 30 years, where treatments have extended and evolved to help both the physical and psychological needs of the patient group. It is particularly useful for pouch patients because some experience a variety of difficult symptoms pertaining specifically to bowel frequency, evacuatory dysfunction and incontinence. This chapter explores some of the techniques employed in Biofeedback which may improve pouch function.

**Keywords** Nurse-led care · Bowel dysfunction · Evacuatory dysfunction Behavioural therapy · Bowel and muscle retraining · Psychological support Lifestyle modification

## 12.1 Introduction

### *12.1.1 Biofeedback Therapy*

The indication for biofeedback is to improve the health of a patient by connecting the influence of the mind with the physiological processes, which in turn develops an enhanced understanding and recognition of activity within the body [1, 2].

Any alterations in the body, poor coping and irrational beliefs may disrupt our aptitude to achieve an essential activity such as bowel function and enforce the distress further [3]. It is biofeedback therapy, the techniques used and having the patient at the centre of any decision making, by developing the relationship as parallel partners, [4] that can help the individual to gain confidence and take control

---

B. Collins (✉) · E. Bradshaw
The Sir Alan Parks Physiology and Neuromodulation Unit, St Marks Hospital, Harrow, Middlesex, UK
e-mail: Brigitte.collins@nhs.net; elissa.bradshaw@nhs.net



J. Warusavitarne, Z. Perry-Woodford (eds.), *The Ileoanal Pouch*,
https://doi.org/10.1007/978-3-319-94385-5_12

of their symptoms and modify learned patterns and behaviours [5, 6]. Developing a therapeutic relationship and promoting effective commitment in treatment may support adherence and compliance to therapy and, definitively, improve symptoms and quality of life [7].

The overall aim of biofeedback therapy in bowel dysfunction, is to attain and maintain a satisfactory bowel pattern and bowel function. It is used in bowel disorders of the lower gastrointestinal tract such as constipation, evacuatory dysfunction and faecal incontinence, and uses education and methods of psychological support, lifestyle modifications, behavioural retraining and re-education of the specific muscles that are used in defaecation [8]. These include the muscles on the lower abdomen and pelvic floor. Biofeedback Therapy can be performed using a variety of techniques including verbal or visual feedback.

The American Neurogastroenterology and Motility Society, the European Society of Neurogastroenterology and Motility, and the Rome IV [9] criteria consider biofeedback therapy to be beneficial for faecal incontinence, irritable bowel syndrome and constipation/evacuation under the configuration of gut-brain interaction [9]. Therefore, it can be seen to apply to some of the symptoms that can be experienced by patients with an ileoanal pouch.

### *12.1.2 Biofeedback and Pouch Function*

The formation of the ileoanal pouch is now the gold standard treatment for many patients with Ulcerative Colitis or Familial Adenomatous Polyposis, whom require colonic removal [10]. The mainstay of Biofeedback is to address the most problematic symptoms for the individual patient and aims to ameliorate these using a multi modal therapy [8]. It is useful for pouch patients who experience a variety of difficult symptoms, pertaining specifically to bowel frequency, incontinence and difficulty initiating or completing pouch evacuation.

## 12.2 Treatments Within the Biofeedback Pouch Pathway at St Marks Hospital

### *12.2.1 Practical Recommendations*

There is no internationally accepted consensus on which practical recommendations biofeedback therapy should include for any specific problem [11]. There remains a dearth of robust randomised control trials that have looked at modalities within "Biofeedback" however it remains a mainstay of conservative management in lower gastrointestinal disorders, being both minimally invasive and low risk. Following an initial advanced assessment appointment, follow up sessions are arranged to monitor progress, support the patient, and offer alternative recommendations if symptoms are responding to management strategies. Time frames for this vary, but at St Marks Hospital the aim is for follow up appointments every 4–6 weeks for up to 6 sessions of treatment.

### 12.2.2 Machine Biofeedback Therapy

A key component of retraining can involve a sensor or probe inserted into the anal canal to display pressure changes; the patient can then respond to the feedback by using appropriate muscle co-ordination [12]. This is a form of visual "feedback" on muscular co-ordination. Several large studies have shown that biofeedback machines are necessary to effectively address evacuatory dysfunction [13]. Inflations and deflations of a balloon placed low in the pouch, establishing newer thresholds for perceptions in the process of emptying can be used to treat rectal hyposensitivity seen in dysynergic defecation [13] and hypersensitivity in faecal urgency.

Similarly a pressure measuring probe can be utilised in retraining pelvic floor muscles. A manometric pressure sensor is placed into the anal canal and patient is asked to voluntarily contract the anal sphincter, high resolution technology shows pressure changes and the patient can respond appropriately to the visual aid.

Treatments are individually tailored to manage the patients' specific needs and expectations. It is important to consider the individuals lifestyle and what is acceptable in terms of management strategies. This can be established through an advanced initial assessment and regular follow up appointments.

### 12.2.3 Education

Including education within the treatment pathway can promote an understanding of the anatomy and physiology of the pelvic floor [14]. Combining this with results of any investigations can significantly increase the individuals understanding of their bowel dysfunction further thus encouraging compliance with treatment [15, 16]. Early management of expectations is key within the field of Biofeedback [18].

### 12.2.4 Optimising Pharmacotherapy

Frequency with pouch patients, in excess of 10 times per day, can be problematic for patients. Most patients would have optimised their dosage of Loperamide to address this, but it is worth re-assessing. Alternative medications such as bile acid sequestrants and maximum doses of Loperamide and codeine may be considered for those troubled by excessive frequency, under the guidance of the medical/surgical and pouch care team [17]. Dosage times can also be changed to ensure doses are taken

30 min prior to any meal, or to incorporate a bigger dose at night to reduce passive nocturnal faecal incontinence.

### *12.2.5 Dietary Modification*

Many pouch patients have self- managed their diet and adhere to a low fibre diet. This advice is reiterated and the patients diet reassessed, suggestions may be made with regard to other basic advice such as reduction of caffeine and artificial sugars which can decrease excessive frequency and faecal leakage for some patients [16].

Ongoing referral to a specialist dietician may also be considered for more complex exclusion diets.

## 12.3 Evacuation Techniques

Evacuatory dysfunction with a difficulty or inability to either initiate and/ or complete bowel evacuation can have either structural and/or functional causes. Inability to empty can be caused by functional problems such as poor co-ordination between abdominal effort and anal relaxation (dyssynergic defaecation) or inability to relax the anal muscles (anismus) [13].

Effective treatment for pouch evacuation includes use of the "brace exercise" which increases intra-abdominal pressure and encourages relaxation of the anal sphincter. Patients are asked to bulge out the lower abdomen using the oblique abdominal muscles to create intra-abdominal pressure. Whilst keeping the abdomen bulged out, the patient pushes towards the anus for 2–3 s, relaxing for a second (keeping the abdomen bulged but not pushing) and repeating this action several times. This technique, can be used to initiate and complete pouch evacuation and avoids excessive straining.

### *12.3.1 Balloon Expulsion*

Pouch evacuation can be assessed by inserting a rectal balloon into the pouch and inflating the balloon via a luer lock syringe, providing the patient with an urge to defaecate. The Biofeedback therapist assesses the patients' balloon expulsion attempt, observing for propulsion breathing and relaxation during the attempt to expel the balloon [12, 13]. Many patients demonstrate poor propulsion or paradoxical contraction [12, 13]. The balloon can be used to teach appropriate use of intra-abdominal pressure and propulsive effort. The balloon technique provides a way of re-educating the patient to use correct defaecatory dynamics through verbal and sensory feedback.

### *12.3.2 Urge Resistance/Pouch Compliance*

Similarly, the rectal balloon may be used in "urge resistance training" for patients with faecal urgency and urge incontinence. Patients can learn to resist the urge and retrain pouch responses accordingly, noting that control can be taken allowing for the urgency to abate. Adopting such techniques validates how in a real life situation, if stools have some form, the urgency can dissipate, demonstrating that the patients will often be able to defer defaecation with pouch compliance training.

### *12.3.3 Sphincter and Pelvic Floor Exercises*

Pelvic floor muscle exercises have been found to significantly reduce anal incontinence [18]. Regular exercises of the anal sphincter, pelvic floor and accessory muscles will tone and increase muscle fibres [18]. Both pelvic muscle exercises and machine sensor biofeedback can improve symptoms of urgency and incontinence by improving contraction of pelvic floor muscles, the motor coordination required for continence, and the perception of pouch distension [18].

### *12.3.4 Neuromuscular Stimulation*

Biofeedback and electrical stimulation may enhance the outcome of treatment compared to anal sphincter exercises alone [11, 13]. Very limited evidence means that any conclusions drawn from current research are at best tentative [11]. In our experience neuromuscular stimulation can be very helpful to patients augmenting the results of their home exercises and improving their sensation. Patients feel the electrical involuntary muscle contraction, which can assist in learning how to contract muscles actively [11] Optimal muscle stimulation should involve a frequency of 40–50 Hz, impulses lasting 5 s, and 5-s pauses to allow the muscle to rest, and occur for approximately 20 min [11].

### *12.3.5 Medena Catheters and Irrigation*

There is very little clinical evidence for the use of Medena catheters to drain or irrigate the pouch but this can be an effective treatment for those with outflow obstruction [19]. Many patients find this an effective treatment using water irrigation via the catheter. Most recently we have also used the Qufora mini irrigation system as a method of instilling water to address outflow obstruction and for some this provides an acceptable way of initiating and completing pouch emptying.

### 12.3.6 Containment and Skincare

Advice can be given on use of anal inserts or an anal plug to prevent passive leakage from the pouch. This method of containment seems to work well with passive nocturnal faecal incontinence. Where leakage cannot be prevented, advice on skincare using barrier or emollient creams can be given.

### 12.3.7 Psychological Support

The effect of acute and chronic stress on bowel function is acknowledged, if not fully understood [21]. Finding ways to alleviate stress may be recommended and may include relaxation, breathing techniques, meditation [22] along with hypnosis and reframing negative beliefs.

The therapeutic relationship between the patient and biofeedback therapist is pivotal to the success of treatment in terms of providing the support that encourages compliance [18, 24]. Transference or counter transference may occur within the consultation, due to the emotional nature of discussing a topic which may be difficult or embarrassing [18].

The most important factor appears to be the relationship between the therapist and the patient [24]. Increasingly in current practice the individual biofeedback therapist is a hybrid practitioner (34) signifying that the therapist needs to be therapeutic for both physical and psychological conditions. Should the psychological provision be beyond the scope of practice of the biofeedback therapist, a specialist counsellor within the team, is introduced to support the patient. Biofeedback presents options for non- invasive yet effective pouch management strategies employed to manage select symptoms related to pouch dysfunction and improve quality of life.

## 12.4 Summary of Recommendations for Pouch Patients

- Education
- Optimising Pharmacotherapy
- Dietary modification
- Brace Exercise
- Balloon expulsion
- Urge resistance/Pouch compliance
- Pelvic Floor Muscle Exercises
- Irrigation
- Containment
- Psychological support

## References


1. Frank DL, Kershid L, Kiffer JF, Moravec CS, McKee MG. Biofeedback in medicine, who, when, why and how? Ment Health Fam Med. 2010;7(2):85–91.
2. Bailboff BD, Frese MP, Rapgay L. Mind/Body psychological treatments for irritable bowel syndrome. Evid Based Compliment Alternat Med. 2008;5(1):41–50.
3. Zuckerman MJ, Guerra LG, Drossman DA, Foland JA, Gregory GG. Health care seeking behaviours related to bowel complaints. Hispanic versus non-Hispanics whites. Dig Dis Sci. 1996;41(1):77–82.
4. Wiener N. Cybernetics, or control and communication in the animal and the machine. Kessinger Publishing, LLC, Massachusetts, USA; 2007.
5. Siever D. History of biofeedback and neurofeedback. Biofeedback. 2008;36(2):74–81.
6. Brown B. New mind, new body-biofeedback: new directions for the mind. New York: Harper and Row; 1974.
7. Duncan J. IBD, psychosocial functioning and the role of the nurses. In: Psychological Aspects of Inflammatory Bowel Disease, A biopsychosocial approach. New York: Routledge; 2015.
8. Burch J, Collins B. Using biofeedback to treat constipation, faecal incontinence and other bowel disorders. Nurs Times. 2010;106(37):18–20.
9. Drossman DA. Functional gastrointestinal disorders: history, pathophysiology, clinical features, and Rome IV. Gastroenterology. 2016;150(6):1262–79.
10. Lee Kong S, Kiran SP. Ongoing challenges and controversies in ulcerative colitis surgery. Expert Rev Gastroenterol Hepatol. 2016;10(2):187–91.
11. Norton C, Cody J. Biofeedback and/or sphincter exercises for the treatment of faecal incontinence in adults. Cochrane Database Syst Rev. 2012.
12. Bharucha AE, Fletcher JG. Recent advances in assessing anorectal structure and functions. Gastroenterology. 2007;133:1069–74.
13. Cadeddu F, Salis F, De Luca E, Ciangola I, Milito G. Efficacy of biofeedback plus transanal stimulation in the management ofpelvic floor dyssynergia: a randomized trial. Tech Coloproctol. 2015;19(6):333–8. Epub 2015 Mar 6.
14. Ward J. How to educate patients. Gastroenterol Clin North Am. 2011;36:687–711. x.
15. Caress AL. Giving information to patients. Nurs Stand. 2003;17(43):47–54.
16. Swan E. The nurse's role in bowel awareness. Nurs Times. 2002;98(14):42–3.
17. British National Formulary (BNF) 72 (September 2016) Published jointly by BMJ Publishing Group Ltd and Royal Pharmaceutical Society.
18. Horvath A. The therapeutic relationship: From transference to alliance. J Clin Psychol. 2000;56(2):163–73.
19. Perry-Woodford Z, McLaughin S. Ileoanal pouch dysfunction and the use of Medena Catheter following hospital discharge. Br J Community Nurs. 2009;14(11):502–6.
21. Whitehead W, Crowell M, Robinson J, Heller B, Schuster M. Effects of stressful life events on bowel symptoms: subjects with irritable bowel syndrome compared with subjects without bowel dysfunction. Gut. 1992;33:825–30.
22. Seong-Hi P, Keum S, Chang-Bum K. Relaxation Therapy for Irritable Bowel Syndrome: A Systematic Review. Asian Nurs Res. 2014;8(3):182–92.
24. Collins B, Norton C. Managing passive incontinence and incomplete evacuation. Br J Nurs. 2013;22:575–9.

# Chapter 13
# The Kock Pouch (Continent Ileostomy)

**Bruce D. George and Richard Guy**

**Abstract** The Kock pouch procedure is an operation to construct a continent ileostomy which the patient self- catheterises several times a day. The procedure is not widely performed owing to the technical difficulty and the high complication rate associated with the procedure but there is renewed interest in this technique for patients with a failed ileoanal pouch or where an ileoanal pouch is not an option. Patient motivation and expectation must be considered in the preoperative phase as the Kock pouch requires significant patient engagement. This chapter highlights the selection, techniques, post-operative care and complications associated with the Kock pouch.

**Keywords** Continent ileostomy · Internal reservoir · Patient motivation
Complication management · Quality of life

## 13.1 Introduction

The Kock pouch (KP) procedure is an operation to construct a continent ileostomy, which the patient self-catheterises several times a day. The concept of a continent ileostomy was developed by Nils Kock in the late 1960's as an alternative to a standard (incontinent) ileostomy principally for patients with ulcerative colitis (UC). At this time ileostomies had an evil reputation despite Brooke's description of a spouted stoma in 1952 mainly due the poor adhesion of cumbersome appliances and frequent leakages. Kock's original technique [1], which did not include a valve mechanism, involved creating a reservoir from ileum and a short efferent limb which the patient catheterised regularly to empty the reservoir.

The technique was soon modified to create a continent valve by intussuscepting a segment of ileum in the efferent limb towards the reservoir (Fig. 13.1). The Kock pouch gained popularity mainly in Scandinavia but was soon overshadowed by the

B. D. George (✉) · R. Guy
Oxford University Hospitals NHS Foundation Trust, Oxford, UK
e-mail: Bruce.George@ouh.nhs.uk

 
J. Warusavitarne, Z. Perry-Woodford (eds.), *The Ileoanal Pouch*,
https://doi.org/10.1007/978-3-319-94385-5_13

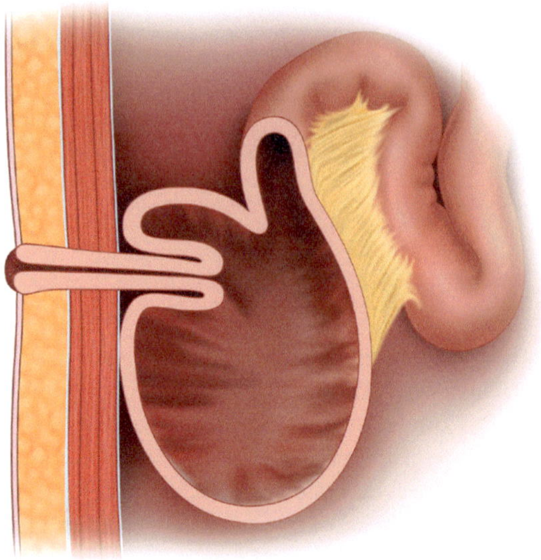

**Fig. 13.1** Diagram of Kock pouch. (Courtesy of Dr. T Oresland)

pelvic ileal pouch-anal anastomosis (IPAA) procedure [2] which rapidly became the gold standard reconstructive option for patients requiring surgery for UC and Familial adenomatous polyposis (FAP). The Kock pouch is now rarely performed outside Sweden and major North American centres and has a reputation for technical complexity, high complication and re-operation rates. There has been recent renewed interest in the Kock pouch technique, driven significantly by patient groups, as an option after failed ileo-anal pouch surgery or in situations where conventional ileo-anal pouch surgery is not appropriate.

## 13.2 Indications (Table 13.1)

Kock pouch (KP) reconstruction is principally indicated in patients with UC either as a salvage after an unsuccessful IPAA or in situations where IPAA is not an option. This includes patients with sphincter damage/incontinence, peri-anal sepsis or UC associated with a low rectal carcinoma. KP may also be undertaken in patients with a previous anus excising pan-proctocolectomy and permanent ileostomy.

The technique may also be considered in analogous situations in FAP.

Crohn's disease is a relative contraindication, although KP reconstruction may be reasonably considered if the Crohn's is isolated to the large bowel. Following proctocolectomy for large bowel Crohn's disease our own preference is to use the "test of time" for about 5 years to ensure no small bowel disease.

The most critical consideration when considering the option of KP surgery is the patient's psychology. The patient needs to be mentally robust as complications/

**Table 13.1** Indications for Kock Pouch reconstruction

| |
|---|
| Ulcerative colitis<br>  When IPAA not an option<br>    Poor sphincters/incontinence<br>    Perianal sepsis<br>    Low rectal carcinoma<br>  Salvage after IPAA<br>  Previous panproctocolectomy and ileostomy |
| Familial adenomatous polyposis (FAP) |
| Crohn's colitis with no evidence of small bowel involvement for >5 years |

re-operations rates are significant and must be prepared to engage significantly in the post-operative care. A patient struggling with a poor quality (flush/leaking) ileostomy should have revision of the stoma before any consideration of KP surgery.

The starting point for most patients when considering KP surgery is likely to be an end ileostomy. In 423 KP patients from the Cleveland Clinic [3], the indications were:

- conversion of end ileostomy to KP (59%)
- total proctocolectomy (20%)
- conversion of failed IPAA to KP (16%)
- completion proctectomy (5%)

## 13.3 Contraindications

The main contraindications are small bowel Crohn's disease and psychological difficulties engaging in the surgery. Patients who are unable to accept the risks of complications and revisional surgery should not undergo KP surgery. Patients with perceived inability to intubate the pouch due to poor eyesight, manual dexterity or mentally unprepared should not undergo KP surgery.

It is important for surgeons and specialist nurses to meet potential patients on several occasions and to liaise closely with their primary care physicians and previous surgical teams.

Relative contraindications are obesity and marginal small bowel length.

## 13.4 **Technique** (Figs. 13.2, 13.3, 13.4, 13.5, and 13.6)

Four distinct stages are recognised:

- Measurement and construction of posterior wall of pouch
- Nipple valve formation and fixation
- Completion of pouch construction

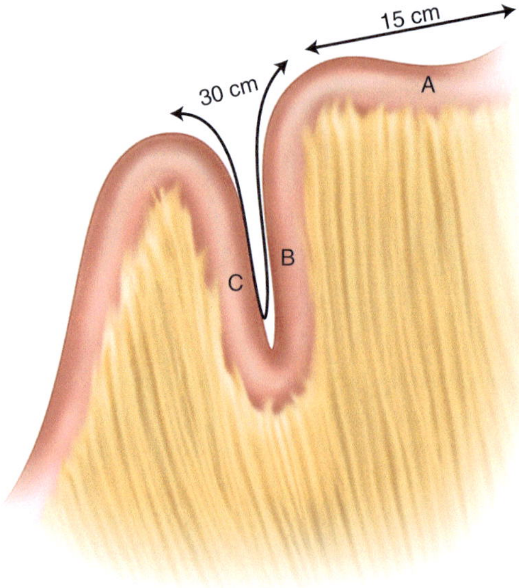


**Fig. 13.2** Measurement of distal 45 cm of ileum

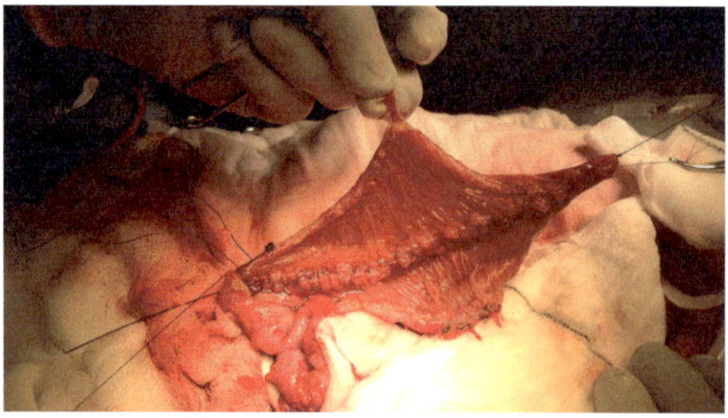

**Fig. 13.3** Opening of anti-mesenteric border of segments B and C + suturing of posterior wall

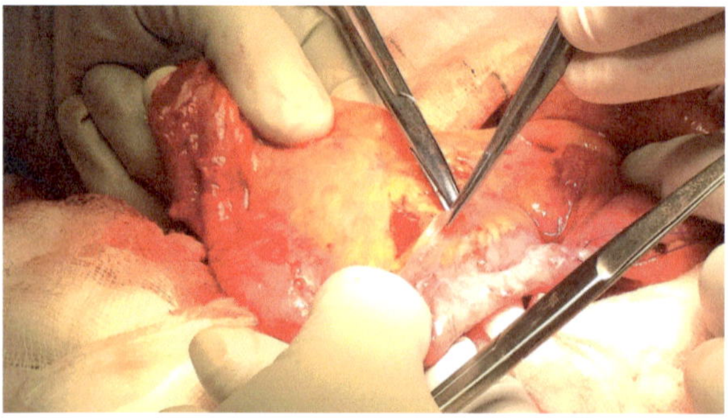

**Fig. 13.4** Striping of visceral peritoneum off segment to be intussuscepted

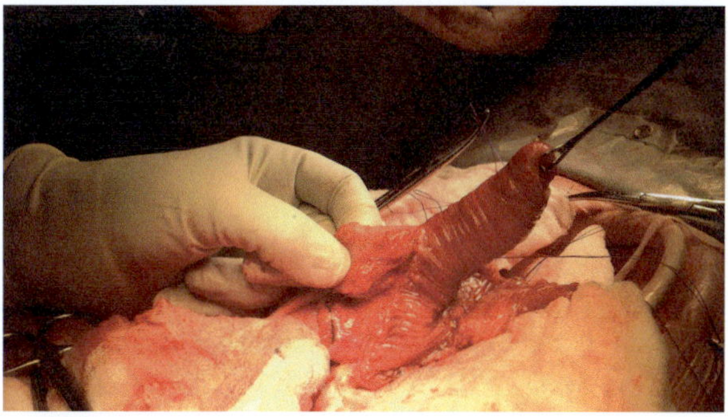

**Fig. 13.5** Intussusception of segment A ileum towards pouch to create valve

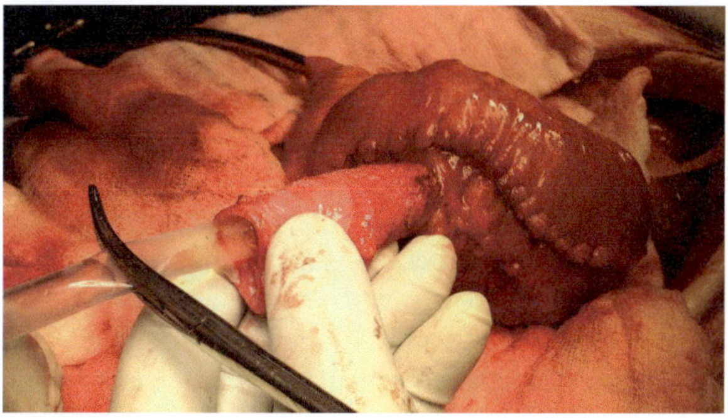

**Fig. 13.6** Insertion of Medena catheter through valve into pouch and testing of integrity

- Stoma formation and fixation of pouch to abdominal wall
- *Measurement and construction of posterior wall of pouch*
  - Three 15 cm bowel segments are marked from the end of the ileum with sutures – the terminal 15 cm (segment A) will be used for the valve and efferent drainage limb, and the two more proximal 15 cm segments (B and C) will form the pouch reservoir (Fig. 13.2).
  - the bowel is opened along the anti-mesenteric border of segments B and C with electrocautery
  - the back walls are apposed and an additional 2 cm should be opened on the antimesenteric border of the afferent end (Fig. 13.3)
  - the back walls are then sutured continuously with a single-layer full-thickness technique using a 4/0 absorbable monofilament suture, the suture on the afferent limb starting at the level of termination of the initial electrocautery cut (the free 2 cm will be used for the start of closure of the anterior pouch wall) (Fig. 13.3).
- *Nipple valve construction and fixation*
  - The nipple valve is constructed by intussuscepting and fixing a segment of small bowel within segment A. A preliminary step is to strip off a triangle of peritoneum over the mesentery of both sides of the efferent limb to be used for the valve is removed (Fig. 13.4), carefully avoiding the underlying vessels –

the purpose of this manoeuvre is to create 'sticky' opposing surfaces to reduce the chance of valve slippage.
  - the efferent limb is intussuscepted towards the pouch by grasping it from within the pouch using a Babcock forceps, aiming for a nipple valve of around 3-5 cm in length (Fig. 13.5)
  - the intussuscepted valve is then fixed in position by firing 3 or 4 non-cutting linear staplers, carefully avoiding the small bowel mesentery
  - external seromuscular 'fundoplication' of the intussusception with several (at least 5) interrupted absorbable sutures also helps to prevent valve slippage

- *Completion of pouch construction*
  - The anterior wall of the pouch is then closed "transversely" to create a more spherical pouch with a running suture using two running seromuscular 4/0 absorbable monofilament sutures making sure the mucosa is inverted; these sutures should start at the apex of the additional 2 cm cut on the afferent limb (Fig. 13.6).
  - the completed pouch, which has a 'banana' shape at this point is flipped to convert it to a rounder configuration. This is difficult to describe but easy to appreciate once seen [4]
  - a 30F Medena catheter is passed through the efferent limb and valve into the pouch and the pouch filled with air via a syringe, clamping the catheter to check for pouch integrity; withdrawal of the catheter from the filled pouch then allows checking the continence of the valve.

- *Stoma formation and fixation of pouch to abdominal wall*
  - A muscle-splitting 1–2 finger diameter trephine is made through the abdominal wall at a site marked pre-operatively by a stomatherapist familiar with Kock pouch management; siting is usually lower than with a conventional ileostomy and a location near to bony prominences may not be such a problem in view of the omission of an external appliance
  - the pouch is orientated to lie anatomically and four spaced interrupted 2/0 monofilament absorbable sutures are placed, picking up anterior rectus sheath and the pouch at the level of the cuff on lateral and medial aspects of the pouch
  - the efferent limb is passed through the abdominal wall ensuring that the pouch has not been twisted, and the pre-placed sutures are tied, ensuring that the cuff sits at the level of the abdominal wall just within the inner part of the trephine; additional sutures are then placed from within to ensure that the pouch sits secure and snug against the abdominal wall
  - following maturation of the stoma, with the abdomen still open, the Medena catheter should be passed into the pouch to ensure straightforward intubation and the pouch test-inflated once more

– the stoma is then matured flush at skin level with an interrupted absorbable 3/0 multifilament suture; the catheter is reinserted into the pouch and marked at stoma level with indelible ink or suture, and is then secured to the abdominal skin with two separately placed sutures wrapped securely around the catheter to prevent dislodgement
– the abdomen is closed, the wound dressed and the Medena catheter (ideally a curved variety) further secured with tape over a bandage roll placed on the lateral side of the stoma, allowing the catheter to drain freely into a drainage bag over the side of the bed

In most situations, a defunctioning proximal loop ileostomy is not undertaken as this would create a high output stoma with associated problems. Optimum management however does depend on prolonged catheter drainage of the pouch in the early post-operative period.

## 13.5 Post-operative Care

The Medena catheter should remain in place on free drainage for 14 days 24 h a day. This is to prevent obstruction and to avoid pouch distension. The catheter should be flushed using the following regime:

- first 24 h – flush every 4 h with 20–30 ml sterile saline
- after 24 h – flush every 6 h, and when needed, for 14 days
- after 3 days tap water may be used for flushing
- check the catheter frequently once the patient starts eating ensuring that it doesn't block
- if the catheter blocks, gently flush the catheter and, if necessary, rotate or milk the catheter until it runs freely

During the first 2 weeks, the patient should be on a low residue diet.

After 14 days, the patient is instructed in catheter changes with the stoma care nurse and the following regime is undertaken:

- day 14–20 the catheter is plugged during the day and the plug removed every hour for flushing, and during the night is connected to a drainage bag
- day 21–27 the plug is removed every 2 h, and at night connected to a drainage bag
- day 28, the catheter is removed completely
- during the 5th week, the pouch is emptied every 3 h and once at night, and should be flushed 3–4 times a day depending on consistency of output

Once the patient is confident in the use of the Medena catheter he/she is discharged to outpatient follow-up under close supervision of the stomatherapy and surgical teams. It should be possible to place a simple swab and adherent dressing over the stoma site between catheterisations.

## 13.6 Complications

The potential complications of this procedure are broadly similar to those after any major gastrointestinal operation. Specific problems after KP surgery are discussed in this section.

The most common early problem is ensuring correct positioning and patency of the draining Medena catheter. Regular flushing and a low residue diet as outlined above is important. If the catheter falls out it should be carefully re-inserted by a surgeon or specialist nurse familiar with the procedure. If difficult to re-intubate this may be undertaken safely with endoscopic/guidewire assistance.

The most feared early complication is leakage from the pouch or efferent limb/valve area. The most vulnerable area is the anterior pouch closure line close to the intussuscepted valve. Leakage rates of around 7% are reported and may require re-operation, repair and probably de-functioning,

Acute complications, such as sepsis, anastomotic or suture-line leaks, stomal ischaemia and intubation difficulty are likely to require a combination of imaging modalities depending upon priorities, clinical suspicion and imaging availability. Cross-sectional (CT or MRI) imaging, for example, supplemented by water-soluble contrast instillation of the pouch, is likely to be most sensitive for the diagnosis of leaks, early fistulas and peri-pouch collections. Early endoscopic examination of the stoma and pouch may be indicated in the case of stomal ischaemia or infarction but this should proceed with caution using a gastroscope and minimal insufflation (with carbon dioxide) for fear of perforation. Careful endoscopic examination may need to be undertaken under general anaesthesia in the event of early difficulties with intubation.

Later major problems with Kock pouches are mainly technical, especially related to the nipple valve, particularly slippage, which is largely responsible for the high reoperation rates. Significant specific complications include:

- nipple valve slippage/prolapse
- dislocation of pouch from abdominal wall
- fistula
- stomal stricture
- pouchitis

### 13.6.1 Valve Problems and Dislocation

Failure of the valve mechanism or dislocation of the pouch from the abdominal wall represent the most challenging complications of this operation. Valve slippage is probably more common in patients with a higher BMI. Most problems occur within the first year of KP construction and most can be corrected with revisional surgery, although a small number of patients become "recurrent offenders" [3].

Typical symptoms of valve problems or pouch dislocation are stoma leakage, increasing difficulty with intubating or overt prolapse. Patients with poor KP function or symptoms of valve displacement should undergo endoscopic and/or radiological assessment. Where catheterisation of the valve is difficult, general anaesthesia and endoscopic guidance may be required. An indwelling catheter may stabilise a faulty valve in the short term.

The majority of patients with valve failure require major revisional surgery. In a series of 31 patients undergoing revision after a mean period of 19.7 years (range 11.7–28.2 years), overall KP salvage success rate was 93% with minimal morbidity, and only 2 patients required pouch excision [5]. Some 12 patients (38.7%) required more than one operation, and procedures included "standard" valve reconstruction (abrasion and cauterisation to generate a fibrotic response; re-intussusception; stapler fixation with a bladeless linear stapler; suture reinforcement to maintain the intussusception; injection of sclerosant; suture bolstering of outflow tract to pouch wall), "turnaround" procedures or pedicle repairs (when valves are too short or re-intussusception is impossible), wall stapling and fistula repair. KP patients may be highly motivated having developed a strong emotional bond with their pouch and will often tolerate multiple revisions if necessary.

### 13.6.2 Fistula

Fistula affecting a KP may arise from the pouch itself, usually from a leak at the suture line, or from the region of the valve. When occurring early after construction, fistulae may settle with conservative management including long-term Medena catheter drainage and appropriate nutritional support. A proximal loop ileostomy may be required. Fistulae involving the valve mechanism are likely to require revisional surgery. Fistulae occurring later may be related to repeated trauma from intubation, but of course raise the question of Crohn's disease.

### 13.6.3 Stricture

Stricturing may occur at stoma level, or at valve level, most likely from ischaemia. Stricturing close to the skin may respond to regular dilatation or a local procedure such as "trimming" of the stenosed end or a local flap such as V-Yplasty. Strictures not amenable to local treatment may require major pouch revision.

### 13.6.4 Pouchitis

Pouchitis is well recognised after KP surgery and probably occurs with a similar frequency to pouchitis after conventional ileo-anal pouch surgery. The management is broadly similar.

## 13.7 Long-Term Durability of Kock Pouch

Nessar [6] reported 10 and 20-year pouch survival rates of 87% and 77%, respectively, in a series of 330 patients over a 27-year period. Such figures compare very favourably with the best IPAA results. Successful retention of a KP depends upon the willingness of the patient and surgeon to embark on revision surgery, possibly many times. Jarvinen [7] reported an early series of 76 patients with a mean follow-up of 9 years, in which revisional surgery was required in 49 patients (66%), mainly for nipple valve failure, and good functional results were ultimately attained in 62 (83%) patients. Similarly, Lepisto [8], during long–term follow–up (mean 18 years) of 96 patients, reported cumulative success rates of 96% at 1 year, 86% at 10 years, 77% at 15 years and 71% at 29 years. Some 85 re-reconstructions were performed among 57 patients (59%), and of these patients 14 had pouch excision. The commonest reasons for pouch excision in these series were recurrent valve dysfunction, fistulas, Crohn's disease and refractory pouchitis.

## 13.8 Quality of Life

Quality of life after KP surgery depends on the "technical" outcome of the surgery but is also critically dependant on the patient's ability to cope with management of the pouch and the need for revisional surgery. Good quality of life (QoL) is reported in many series [8–10]. Patients tend to be highly motivated to retain their continent ileostomy even if multiple revisions are necessary to achieve this. Specific QoL questionnaire assessment, comparing 68 KP patients (median age 60 years at follow-up) with a median follow-up of 31 years with a randomly-selected age-matched and gender-match sample from the Swedish population, showed health-related QoL to be similar in the two groups [11], with 78% of KP patients rating their overall health as "good, very good or excellent".

## 13.9 Conclusions

Kock pouch construction may be considered as an alternative to a traditional ileostomy principally for patients with UC, either after a failed pelvic pouch or in patients in whom a pelvic pouch is not appropriate. The procedure is technically demanding and has a predictably high need for revisional surgery. Patients needs to be carefully selected, psychologically robust and well supported. Similarly, colorectal units offering continent KP reconstruction need to be carefully selected, well trained and robust.

## References


1. Kock NG. Intra-abdominal "reservoir" in patients with permanent ileostomy. Preliminary observations on a procedure resulting in fecal "continence" in five ileostomy patients. Arch Surg. 1969;99:223–31.
2. Parks AG, Nicholls RJ. Proctocolectomy without ileostomy for ulcerative colitis. Br Med J. 1978;2:86–8.
3. Aytac E, Ashburn J, Dietz DW. Is there still a role for continent ileostomy in the treatment of inflammatory bowel disease? Inflamm Bowel Dis. 2014;20:2519–25.
4. Bloemendaal AL, Lovegrove R, Buchs NC, Guy RJ, George BD. Continent ileostomy (Kock pouch) formation – a video vignette. Color Dis. 2017;19:85–6.
5. Denoya PI, Schluender SJ, Bub DS, Gorfine SR, Bauer JJ. Delayed Kock pouch nipple valve failure: is revision indicated? Dis Colon Rectum. 2008;51:1544–7.
6. Nessar G, Fazio VW, Tekkis P, et al. Long-term outcome and quality of life after continent ileostomy. Dis Colon Rectum. 2006;49:336–44.
7. Jarvinen HJ, Makitie A, Sivula A. Long-term results of continent ileostomy. Int J Color Dis. 1986;1:40–3.
8. Lepisto AH, Jarvinen HJ. Durability of Kock continent ileostomy. Dis Colon Rectum. 2003;46:925–8.
9. Lian LF, Fazio V, Dietz D, Remzi F, Shen B, Wu R, et al. Outcomes after conversion of failed ileal pouch-anal anastomosis (IPAA) to continent ileostomy (CI) in a single tertiary center. Dis Colon Rectum. 2008;51:2.
10. Parc Y, Klouche M, Bennis M, Lefevre JH, Shields C, Tiret E. The continent ileostomy: an alternative to end ileostomy? Short and long-term results of a single institution series. Dig Liver Dis. 2011;43:779–83.
11. Berndtsson I, Lindholm E, Oresland T, Hulten L. Health-related quality of life and pouch function in continent ileostomy patients: a 30 year perspective. Dis Colon Rectum. 2004;47:2131–7.

# Chapter 14
# The Ileorectal Anastomosis in Ulcerative Colitis

**Pär Myrelid and Disa Kalman**

**Abstract** The ileoanal pouch has been the accepted restorative procedure for ulcerative colitis but this can be associated with complications and issues related to function. Preserving the rectum has inherent benefits but this has to be weighed against the risk of proctitis and its associated issues. This chapter aims to examine the emerging role of ileorectal anastomosis in ulcerative colitis as an alternative to the ileoanal pouch and describes functional outcomes and prognosis.

**Keywords** Ileorectal anastomosis · Surveillance · Cancer risk · Quality of life Failure

## 14.1 Introduction

Colectomy is still frequently required in the care of ulcerative colitis and up to 30% of patients will have surgery over the course of time [1]. There are conflicting data regarding a possible recent decrease in surgery rates owing to the introduction of biologics in emergency situation combined with immune modulators as maintenance therapy [1–3]. Subtotal colectomies in ulcerative colitis can be divided into emergency procedures or semi-elective procedures. Emergency colectomies are performed in patients with acute severe colitis not responding to medical management, because of the risk of developing life threatening complications such as toxic megacolon, perforation or severe bleeding. Elective colectomies are performed in patients with dysplasia or cancer, chronic colitis refractory to medical management, steroid dependence or intolerance to long term immunomodulation or other medical therapies. Most patients undergoing surgery are quite young and have high expectations of quality of life and a life without ileostomy if possible.

P. Myrelid (✉) · D. Kalman
Department of Surgery, Linköping University Hospital, County Council of Östergötland, Linköping, Sweden

Division of Surgery, Department of Clinical and Experimental Medicine, Faculty of Health Sciences, Linköping University, Linköping, Sweden
e-mail: par.myrelid@liu.se



J. Warusavitarne, Z. Perry-Woodford (eds.), *The Ileoanal Pouch*,
https://doi.org/10.1007/978-3-319-94385-5_14

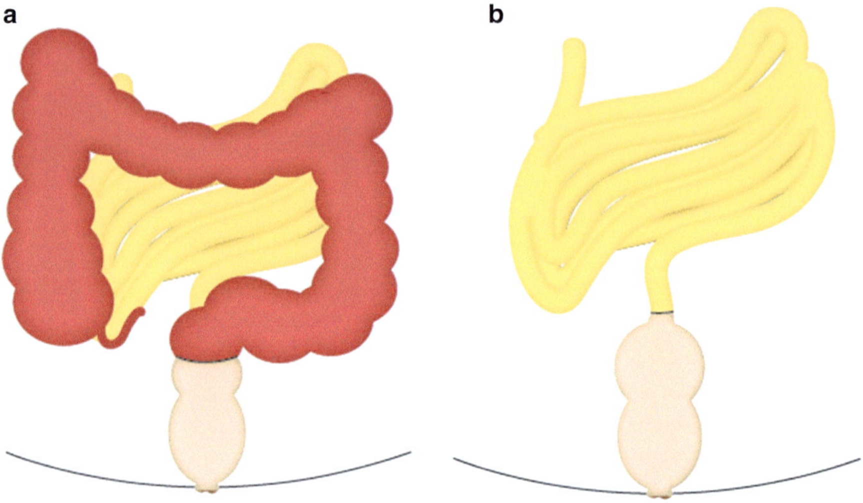


**Fig. 14.1** (**a**) Subtotal colectomy (**b**) Ileo rectal anastomosis

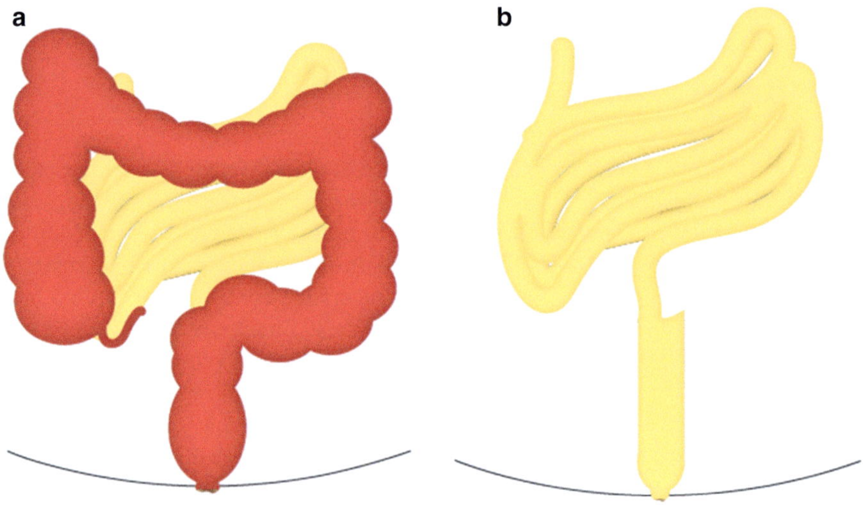


**Fig. 14.2** (**a**) Proctocolectomy as a one- or two stage procedure (**b**) Ileal pouch anal anastomosis

The first described restorative method after colectomy in ulcerative colitis was the ileorectal anastomosis (Fig. 14.1) [4] and later the continent ileostomy was introduced by Nils G Kock [5]. Both these methods were also used as reconstruction after colectomy in the hereditary disease familial adenomatous polyposis (FAP) and in some cases of severe constipation. The use of both these methods decreased in clinical use when the ileal pouch anal anastomosis (Fig. 14.2) became gold standard for both FAP and ulcerative colitis after its introduction by Parks and Nicholls in the

1970's [6–8]. The diminishing use of the Kock pouch was mainly due to the need for revisional surgeries and in the case of ileorectal anastomosis due to recurrent proctitis and risk of rectal cancer in the long run [9]. Lately long term follow up data have shown some problems with the ileal pouch anal anastomosis as well with a yearly failure rate (diversion or excision) of approximately 0.6–1.9%, partly dependent on hospital volumes [10–16]. Topical high dose anti-inflammatory medication together with meticulous endoscopic surveillance has led to the reintroduction of the ileorectal anastomosis in parts of the world, mainly based on reports showing impaired fertility in young patients going through restorative proctocolectomy with ileal pouches [17–21]. Medications have different advantages and disadvantages and so have surgical restorative methods. We aim to shed some light on the ileorectal anastomosis in this context in general, as used in FAP and Crohn's diseases, but mainly focus on its use in ulcerative colitis.

## 14.2 Surgical Procedure

Today, with laparoscopic subtotal colectomy being the standard procedure in ulcerative colitis [22] a laparoscopic approach creating the ileorectal anastomosis is easily performed and in most cases it can be performed as a single incision procedure [23]. The patient is placed in lithotomy position and the end ileostomy is taken down. Before reentering the small bowel end to the abdominal cavity the anvil of a circular stapler is inserted into the open end of the small bowel and secured with a tight purse string. A wound protector is inserted through the stoma opening with a surgical glove wrapped around the outer ring. Two or three ports can thereafter be inserted through the fingers of the surgical glove with an air tight ligature (preferably a rubber ligature or one of the fingers from another surgical glove) around it. After pneumoperitoneum is established the top of the rectum is localized where after the circular stapler is inserted through the anal opening and is brought to the proximal end of the rectum by direct vision from the laparoscopy inside the abdominal cavity. After docking of the anvil to the circular stapling device, but before firing the stapler, the correct localization of the small bowel is assured to ensure no twisting of the ileorectal anastomosis is made. After regular inspection of the two anastomotic doughnuts an air-leak test with fluid in the abdominal cavity and inflating air, as well as looking at the anastomosis, using a rigid or flexible sigmoidoscope. If the anastomosis is satisfactory the wound retractor is removed and the fascia and skin closed in a regular way.

## 14.3 Functional Outcome

One of the main concerns patients have regarding the functional outcome after a reconstruction is the number of bowel movements (day and night), continence and fear of recurrent problems with urgent bowel evacuation. This will be influenced by any ongoing inflammation (proctitis, pouchitis or cuffitis), the volume and compliance of the rectum or the pouch as well as the sensory function [24, 25]. This may differ somewhat between patients with polyposis and ulcerative colitis.

In published reports on both polyposis and ulcerative colitis the number of bowel movements during 24 h range between 3 and 6 for the ileorectal anastomosis [17, 18, 21, 26, 27] compared to 5–7 for the pelvic pouch [28]. The frequency of nocturnal bowel movements has also been studied showing an advantage for the ileorectal anastomosis compared with the pelvic pouch, 13–41% and 53% respectively [18, 28–31] (Table 14.1).

In the case of polyposis the ileorectal anastomosis seems to offer a somewhat better function in comparison with the pelvic pouch in regards of the number of bowel movements, leakages, need for a protective pad, capability to distinguish gas from stool as well as need for dietary restrictions [32]. Comparisons between the ileorectal anastomosis and the pelvic pouch regarding continence has been less studied but in ulcerative colitis compared with FAP. In the latter case Günter et al. showed a significant advantage for the ileorectal anastomosis over the pelvic pouch measured with incontinence scores [29]. Further, polyposis patients do not have the risks of developing proctitis and their function will be more stable over time. Börjesson et al. evaluated the function and continence after restorative surgery in ulcerative colitis in a single unit, comparing ileo-rectal anastomosis and pelvic pouches [24].

**Table 14.1** Advantages and disadvantages of reconstructive methods after colectomy for ulcerative colitis

| Surgical method | Advantages | Disadvantages |
|---|---|---|
| Ileostomy | Seldom need of revision<br>Controlled emtying from stoma bag<br>Preservation of fertility (as long as rectum is left in place) | Negative impact on body image<br>Negative impact on sexual function<br>Uncontrolled emptying into stoma bag<br>Cancer risk (as long as rectum is left in place) |
| Ileorectal anastomosis | Less complicated procedure<br>Transanal defecation<br>Less frequent bowel movements<br>Continence<br>No (or postponed) pelvic surgery<br>Preservation of fertility | Risk of proctitis<br>Need of anti-inflammatory medication<br>Urgencies<br>Need of surveillance<br>Cancer risk |
| Ileal pouch anal anastomosis | Transanal defecation<br>No remaining disease (apart from rectal cuff in stapled anastomoses)<br>Very low risk of cancer | Complicated procedure<br>More frequent bowel movements<br>Impaired continence (especially night time)<br>Risk of pouchitis<br>Impaired sexual function and fecundability |
| Kock's continent ileostomy | Controlled emptying of stoma<br>Patient controlling bowel rather than bowel controlling patient | Need of revisions (locally or abdominal)<br>Risk of pouchitis<br>Complicated procedure (few centers world-wide with contemporary experience) |

They found soiling or need for protective pads to be less frequent among patients with an ileorectal anastomosis, (11%), compared with (28–34%) those who have a pelvic pouch. On the other hand, problems with urgency were more common among patients with an ileorectal anastomosis than a pelvic pouch, (33% and 16% respectively). Urgency after ileorectal anastomosis in ulcerative colitis was also found to be more common than in patients with a pelvic pouch in a report from the Cleveland Clinic [31]. In the same report they also found patients to have less frequent bowel movements and less nightly seepage if they were restored with an ileorectal anastomosis. In a more recent report from a single center in Sweden patients with ileorectal anastomosis (n = 89) reported significantly less bowel movements in comparison with patients with pelvic pouch (n = 108). [17] Some of the advantages and disadvantages of the different procedures are summarized in Table 14.1.

## 14.4 Sexual Function and Fecundity

Sexual function is an important consideration particularly in the IBD population as it often affects young individuals. The effect of reconstructive surgery has been evaluated in FAP. Some studies show a less favorable outcome for pelvic pouch regarding physical and sexual function [33, 34]. This has led some of these authors to advocate ileorectal anastomosis as a first step procedure in young individuals postponing the pelvic pouch until the affected individuals are older and preferably in a long term relationship [33]. Van Balkom et al. reported on young patients (11 males and 15 females) with FAP (n = 10) and ulcerative colitis (n = 16) being reconstructed with pelvic pouch. All the males reported acceptable sexual function while 50% of the females showed signs indicating sexual dysfunction [34]. Similar reports have been published showing sexual dysfunction in almost half of the pelvic pouch patients [35] and just as in the report from van Balkom et al. especially among females [36]. These findings are however quite different from two Scandinavian report advocating a favorable outcome in ulcerative colitis patients having a pelvic pouch [37, 38]. Koivusalo et al. reported 84% satisfactory sexual function and 68% enjoyable sex life in ulcerative colitis patients who had been reconstructed with a pelvic pouch during childhood or adolescence [37]. Fecundity is the actual reproductive rate and often expressed as the fecundability or the probability to conceive in a specific time period. In FAP the fecundability is unchanged after an ileorectal anastomosis and comparable to that of the general population, while it drops to 0.54 ($p = 0.004$) after pelvic pouch [39]. The same findings were seen after pelvic pouch in females with ulcerative colitis where it dropped to 0.20 ($p < 0.0001$) from preoperative rates which were at the same level as within the background population [40]. A meta-analysis showed that the pelvic pouch, regardless of whether performed for FAP or ulcerative colitis, increased the infertility rate from 20% before to 63% after the pelvic pouch [41] (Table 14.1). The mechanism is thought to be occlusion of the Fallopian tubes by pelvic scarring and adhesions [42], which may be more severe in an inflammatory condition like ulcerative colitis compared with FAP.

Three smaller studies including patients from five European expert centers comparing complete laparoscopic and/or hand-assisted laparoscopic pelvic pouch with open procedures found the laparoscopic approach to have less risk of infertility [43–45]. This still needs further evaluation as older and much larger epidemiological nationwide studies have shown such drastic negative effect by a pelvic pouch procedure compared with an IRA, but with no effect by the subtotal colectomy itself [39–41].

## 14.5 Quality of Life

The quality of life in ulcerative colitis is dependent on a range of different factors such as the degree of symptoms (remission or active disease), co-morbidity and gender [46]. Health-related quality of life has been compared between ulcerative colitis patients in remission on anti-TNF therapy and patients reconstructed with pelvic pouch after proctocolectomy. No differences were found regarding health-related quality of life or disability, despite a significantly higher stool frequency and need of anti-diarrheal medication in patients with pelvic pouch [47]. Similarly, in FAP patients pelvic pouch and ileorectal anastomosis had similar outcomes regarding quality of life, despite better function with the ileorectal anastomosis [32]. In the report by Moreira et al. ileorectal anastomosis in ulcerative colitis was associated with fewer bowel movements, less night time seepage but increased urgency compared with the pelvic pouch. Regardless of this, no differences in quality of life was found between the groups apart from some dietary and work restrictions in ileorectal anastomosis [31].

## 14.6 Medication, Cancer Risk and Surveillance

Patients with ulcerative colitis reconstructed with an ileorectal anastomosis have a higher need for anti-inflammatory medication, ranging from 60% to 91% [17, 18, 21, 31] (Table 14.1). Due to the anti-inflammatory effect and a possible cancer preventing effect topical high dose use of 5-ASA medication is often proposed and even considered standard of care in some centers (Table 14.2) [17, 18, 48, 49]. The experience of using immunomodulators and/or biologic medications in ulcerative colitis patients with ileorectal anastomosis is thus far limited, while its role in Crohn's disease is more established [50–52]. In most Swedish units performing ileorectal anastomosis for ulcerative colitis the algorithm so far has been proctectomy and pelvic pouch in patients later developing intractable proctitis despite the use of topical 5-ASA.

The risk of rectal cancer was one of the main reasons for abandoning ileorectal anastomosis after colectomy for ulcerative colitis [9] and the risk of developing rectal cancer needs to be borne in mind (Tables 14.1 and 14.2). However, in several

**Table 14.2** Maintenance therapy and surveillance algorithm for reconstruction with ileorectal anastomosis in ulcerative colitis

| **Medical therapy** | |
|---|---|
| Maintenance therapy is recommended with topical mesalamine 500–1000 mg twice daily | |
| **Surveillance** | |
| Surveillance is recommended using flexible endoscopy and multiple random biopsies (as well as from any suspicious area) | |
| Early onset of the disease (<20 years of age) and <10 years duration: | Yearly interval |
| Early onset of the disease and >10 years duration: | Twice yearly |
| All others: | Yearly interval |

reports on ileorectal anastomosis in ulcerative colitis no patients developed rectal cancer within 10 years of diagnosis [9, 17, 19, 20, 31] and cancer can also existent in the pelvic pouch, albeit to a lesser extent [17, 53]. A recent national cohort found the relative risk of rectal cancer in ileorectal anastomosis to be increased almost ninefold compared without the general population (without a diagnosis of ulcerative colitis) but with an actual risk of only 1.8% after a mean follow up of 8.6 years (range 0.0–45.1). This gives a cumulative risk of 1.6% at 10 years and 5.6% at 20 years follow up [54]. In the same paper patients reconstructed with an ileorectal anastomosis and with concomitant primary sclerosing cholangitis had an almost sixfold increased risk of rectal cancer compared with those without primary sclerosing cholangitis, and this has also been found in a report from France [55]. The major problem with rectal cancer in ileorectal anastomosis has been poor selection of patients (dysplasia or even colon cancer at time of reconstruction) or insufficient surveillance [17, 54, 55]. There are no guidelines regarding surveillance but annual flexible endoscopy with multiple biopsies is recommended [17, 31]. Accordingly, patients with severe dysplasia, history of colonic cancer, primary sclerosing cholangitis or those unwilling to attend surveillance are not suitable candidates for ileorectal anastomosis (Fig. 14.3) [1, 17, 19, 20, 31].

## 14.7 Surgical Risks and Failure

Reconstruction with an ileorectal anastomosis is a limited procedure in comparison with a pelvic pouch and in a recent Swedish report this was shown to be associated with shorter operating time and less blood loss (Table 14.1). After both procedures the risk of any post-operative complications was quite high but there was a significant advantage for ileorectal anastomosis compared with pelvic pouch, 23.8% and 39.9% respectively, and this also held true for more severe complications (Clavien-Dindo ≥3) [17]. Furthermore most patients with a pelvic pouch will have the pouch protected by a proximal loop ileostomy which will require a second operation to reverse the ileostomy. This procedure, although relatively minor, has its inherent complications [17, 56].

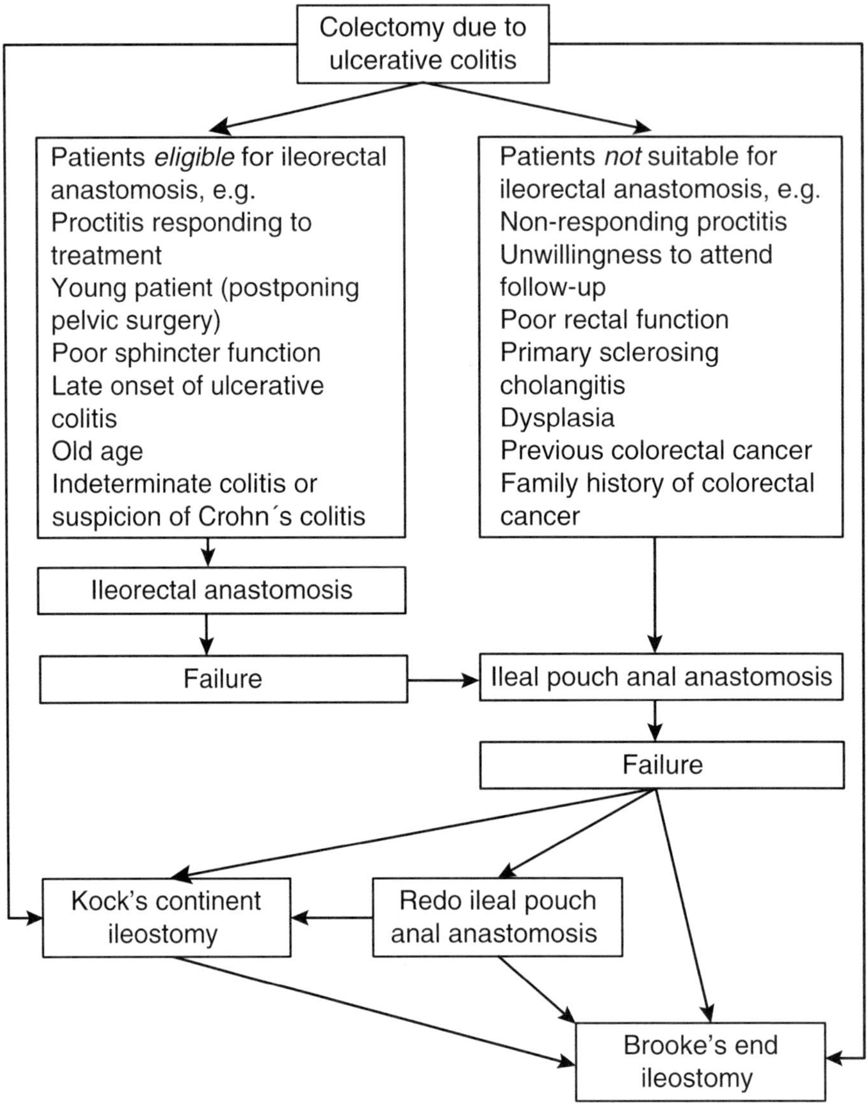


**Fig. 14.3** Possible reconstructive algorithm after colectomy in ulcerative colitis

The need for diversion with a stoma after restorative colectomy, with or without proctectomy or excision of the rectum/pouch in the case of ileorectal anastomosis or pelvic pouch, respectively, is considered a failure. The failure rate for ileorectal anastomosis was 24.1% after 10 years in the latest study by Andersson et al. [17] but seems to be around 16% at 5 years [20, 57] and 31% at 10 years [57, 58]. The failure rate for pelvic pouch is partly dependent on the experience of the team involved in the care of the ulcerative colitis patient [11, 13] and was approximately 1% per year in the UK between 1996 and 2008 [11]. In other reports the failure rate was 6–9% after 5 years and 13–19% after 10 years [15, 17]. In a recent French study patients who had their colectomy due to refractory ulcerative colitis had a significantly worse outcome compared with those who had their colectomy due to acute severe colitis, a hazard ratio of 1.6 having a failure of their IRA [59]. In a similar vein patients naïve to immunomodulators and biologicals before colectomy had a better long term outcome of IRA. Patients with immunomodulators or biologicals had a hazard ratio of failure of 1.3 whereas those with both therapies did even worse with a hazard ration of 2.9 for IRA failure [59].

A possible advantage with the ileorectal anastomosis, if it fails or dysplasia develops, is the chance of performing a proctectomy with a pelvic pouch (Fig. 14.3). About 36–70% of the ulcerative colitis patients with a failed ileorectal anastomosis received a pelvic pouch later on in life [17, 31]. A recent paper on the outcome of such subsequent pelvic pouch found no worse outcome compared with a primary pelvic pouch in regards to failure [60]. There is however limited knowledge regarding the functional outcomes after a subsequent pelvic pouch in ulcerative colitis but in FAP the functional outcome was no worse after a subsequent pelvic pouch compared with a primary [61]. There is of course the possibility of performing a redo of a pelvic pouch the success rates are far from excellent, especially when performed for septic complications, and with much worse function compared with primary pelvic pouches [58, 62].

Comparing the outcomes of ileorectal anastomosis in FAP ulcerative colitis may not always be effective as the latter has an inherent risk of proctitis. However, a meta-analysis comparing pelvic pouch in ulcerative colitis and FAP showed the risk for pouchitis to be higher in ulcerative colitis as well as a small increased stool frequency but with otherwise comparable outcomes in function and failure as in those with FAP [63].

## 14.8 Summary

Colectomy, despite the pharmaceutical evolution in inflammatory bowel disease still a quite frequent procedure in the lifetime of patients with ulcerative colitis.

As medications have different advantages and disadvantages, so have surgical reconstructive methods after a colectomy. The use of ileorectal anastomosis in FAP has been well characterized but the use in ulcerative colitis has been less well described. Despite the lack of complete knowledge recent data have shown that the ileorectal anastomosis, in combination with topical treatment and surveillance, is a safe procedure in ulcerative colitis and with a functional outcome and failure rate well in line with the pelvic pouch. In parts of the world the ileorectal anastomosis has been just as common as the pelvic pouch. Of 994 ulcerative colitis patients undergoing colectomy in Sweden during the period 2000–2010 the reconstructive method was ileorectal anastomosis in 478 cases (48.0%), pelvic pouch in 497 cases (50.0%) and the remaining 19 patients was reconstructed with a continent ileostomy [64]. A randomized controlled trial in Sweden, randomizing between ileorectal anastomosis and pelvic pouch as primary reconstruction in eligible patients after colectomy for ulcerative colitis, was not able to enroll patients due to strong patient opinions after receiving information from surgeons regarding the possible advantages and disadvantages of the two procedures. In Sweden the use of ileorectal anastomosis has mainly been offered to patients with a distensible rectum and good response to topical 5-ASA therapy after subtotal colectomy and without a history of colorectal cancer or high grade dysplasia [17]. Further, patients with primary sclerosing cholangitis or a family history of colorectal cancer are less suitable for ileorectal anastomosis [17, 49, 54, 55], both due to increased risk of cancer and in the former case as well as poor function [65]. Similarly patients with acute severe colitis naïve to more potent medical therapy seems better suited than those with refractory colitis and previous medication with immunomodulators and/or biologicals [59].

Young patients on the other hand could have a favorable outcome with an ileorectal anastomosis, possibly as a temporary solution, with regard to fecundity and sexual function. Furthermore, patients with an onset of the late disease in life and/or a short history of colitis could be suitable candidates for ileorectal anastomosis.

The use of ileorectal anastomosis in ulcerative colitis is safe and with acceptable outcomes related to function and risk of failure. It can, in selected cases be used as a permanent solution and in other cases, similar to FAP, as a temporary solution resorting to proctectomy and pelvic pouch later in life. With the use of ileorectal anastomosis as a complement to the continent ileostomy and the ileal pouch anal anastomosis we can increase the choices for patients needing colectomy. Patients with UC or FAP should be introduced to the different choices, their advantages as well as their limitations.

## References

1. Aratari A, Papi C, Clemente V, et al. Colectomy rate in acute severe ulcerative colitis in the infliximab era. Dig Liver Dis. 2008;40:821–6.
2. Kaplan GG, Seow CH, Ghosh S, et al. Decreasing colectomy rates for ulcerative colitis: a population-based time trend study. Am J Gastroenterol. 2012;107:1879–87.
3. Reich KM, Chang HJ, Rezaie A, et al. The incidence rate of colectomy for medically refractory ulcerative colitis has declined in parallel with increasing anti-TNF use: a time-trend study. Aliment Pharmacol Ther. 2014;40:629–38.
4. Aylett SO. Conservative surgery in the treatment of ulcerative colitis. Br Med J. 1953;2:1348–51.
5. Kock NG. Intra-abdominal "reservoir" in patients with permanent ileostomy. Preliminary observations on a procedure resulting in fecal "continence" in five ileostomy patients. Arch Surg. 1969;99:223–31.
6. Parks AG, Nicholls RJ. Proctocolectomy without ileostomy for ulcerative colitis. Br Med J. 1978;2:85–8.
7. McGuire BB, Brannigan AE, O'Connell PR. Ileal pouch-anal anastomosis. Br J Surg. 2007;94:812–23.
8. McLaughlin SD, Clark SK, Tekkis PP, et al. Review article: restorative proctocolectomy, indications, management of complications and follow-up--a guide for gastroenterologists. Aliment Pharmacol Ther. 2008;27:895–909.

9. Baker WN, Glass RE, Ritchie JK, et al. Cancer of the rectum following colectomy and ileorectal anastomosis for ulcerative colitis. Br J Surg. 1978;65:862–8.
10. Andersson P, Norblad R, Söderholm JD, et al. Ileorectal anastomosis in comparison with ileal pouch anal anastomosis in reconstructive surgery for ulcerative colitis--a single institution experience. J Crohns Colitis. 2014;8:582–9.
11. Burns EM, Bottle A, Aylin P, et al. Volume analysis of outcome following restorative proctocolectomy. Br J Surg. 2011;98:408–17.
12. Hahnloser D, Pemberton JH, Wolff BG, et al. Results at up to 20 years after ileal pouch–anal anastomosis for chronic ulcerative colitis. Br J Surg. 2007;94:333–40.
13. Kennedy ED, Rothwell DM, Cohen Z, et al. Increased experience and surgical technique lead to improved outcome after ileal pouch-anal anastomosis: a population-based study. Dis Colon Rectum. 2006;49:958–65.
14. Hueting WE, Buskens E, van der Tweel I, et al. Results and complications after ileal pouch anal anastomosis: a meta-analysis of 43 observational studies comprising 9,317 patients. Dig Surg. 2005;22:69–79.
15. Tulchinsky H, Hawley PR, Nicholls J. Long-term failure after restorative proctocolectomy for ulcerative colitis. Ann Surg. 2003;238:229–34.
16. MacRae HM, McLeod RS, Cohen Z, et al. Risk factors for pelvic pouch failure. Dis Colon Rectum. 1997;40:257–62.
17. Andersson P, Norblad R, Söderholm JD, et al. Ileorectal anastomosis in comparison with ileal pouch anal anastomosis in reconstructive surgery for ulcerative colitis – a single institution experience. J Crohns Colitis. 2014;8(7):582–9. https://doi.org/10.1016/j.crohns.2013.11.014.
18. Börjesson L, Lundstam U, Öresland T, et al. The place for colectomy and ileorectal anastomosis: a valid surgical option for ulcerative colitis? Tech Coloproctol. 2006;10:237–41. discussion 241
19. Mann CV. Total colectomy and ileorectal anastomosis for ulcerative colitis. World J Surg. 1988;12:155–9.
20. Pastore RL, Wolff BG, Hodge D. Total abdominal colectomy and ileorectal anastomosis for inflammatory bowel disease. Dis Colon Rectum. 1997;40:1455–64.
21. Gallone L, Olmi L, Marchetti V. Use of topical rectal therapy to preserve the rectum in surgery of ulcerative colitis. World J Surg. 1980;4:609–13.
22. Oresland T, Bemelman WA, Sampietro GM, et al. European evidence based consensus on surgery for ulcerative colitis. J Crohns Colitis. 2015;9:4–25.
23. Naqi SA, Smyth J, Mortensen N, et al. Single-incision laparoscopic ileorectal anastomosis. Color Dis. 2014;16:O297–9.
24. Öresland T, Fasth S, Nordgren S, et al. The clinical and functional outcome after restorative proctocolectomy. A prospective study in 100 patients. Int J Color Dis. 1989;4:50–6.
25. Öresland T, Fasth S, Nordgren S, et al. Pouch size: the important functional determinant after restorative proctocolectomy. Br J Surg. 1990;77:265–9.
26. Elton C, Makin G, Hitos K, et al. Mortality, morbidity and functional outcome after ileorectal anastomosis. Br J Surg. 2003;90:59–65.
27. da Luz MA, Lavery IC. Ileorectal anastomosis and proctocolectomy with end ileostomy for ulcerative colitis. Clin Colon Rectal Surg. 2010;23:269–73.
28. de Zeeuw S, Ahmed Ali U, Donders RA, et al. Update of complications and functional outcome of the ileo-pouch anal anastomosis: overview of evidence and meta-analysis of 96 observational studies. Int J Color Dis. 2012;27:843–53.
29. Gunther K, Braunrieder G, Bittorf BR, et al. Patients with familial adenomatous polyposis experience better bowel function and quality of life after ileorectal anastomosis than after ileoanal pouch. Color Dis. 2003;5:38–44.
30. Parc R, Legrand M, Frileux P, et al. Comparative clinical results of ileal-pouch anal anastomosis and ileorectal anastomosis in ulcerative colitis. Hepato-Gastroenterology. 1989;36:235–9.
31. da Luz MA, Kiran RP, Lavery I. Clinical outcomes of ileorectal anastomosis for ulcerative colitis. Br J Surg. 2010;97:65–9.

32. Ko CY, Rusin LC, Schoetz DJ Jr, et al. Does better functional result equate with better quality of life? Implications for surgical treatment in familial adenomatous polyposis. Dis Colon Rectum. 2000;43:829–35. discussion 835-7
33. Andrews L, Mireskandari S, Jessen J, et al. Impact of familial adenomatous polyposis on young adults: quality of life outcomes. Dis Colon Rectum. 2007;50:1306–15.
34. van Balkom KA, Beld MP, Visschers RG, et al. Long-term results after restorative proctocolectomy with ileal pouch-anal anastomosis at a young age. Dis Colon Rectum. 2012;55:939–47.
35. Ogilvie JW Jr, Goetz L, Baxter NN, et al. Female sexual dysfunction after ileal pouch-anal anastomosis. Br J Surg. 2008;95:887–92.
36. Larson DW, Davies MM, Dozois EJ, et al. Sexual function, body image, and quality of life after laparoscopic and open ileal pouch-anal anastomosis. Dis Colon Rectum. 2008;51:392–6.
37. Koivusalo A, Pakarinen MP, Natunen J, et al. Sexual functions in adulthood after restorative proctocolectomy for paediatric onset ulcerative colitis. Pediatr Surg Int. 2009;25:881–4.
38. Berndtsson I, Öresland T, Hultén L. Sexuality in patients with ulcerative colitis before and after restorative proctocolectomy: a prospective study. Scand J Gastroenterol. 2004;39:374–9.
39. Olsen KO, Juul S, Bulow S, et al. Female fecundity before and after operation for familial adenomatous polyposis. Br J Surg. 2003;90:227–31.
40. Ording Olsen K, Juul S, Berndtsson I, et al. Ulcerative colitis: female fecundity before diagnosis, during disease, and after surgery compared with a population sample. Gastroenterology. 2002;122:15–9.
41. Rajaratnam SG, Eglinton TW, Hider P, et al. Impact of ileal pouch-anal anastomosis on female fertility: meta-analysis and systematic review. Int J Color Dis. 2011;26:1365–74.
42. Öresland T, Palmblad S, Ellstrom M, et al. Gynaecological and sexual function related to anatomical changes in the female pelvis after restorative proctocolectomy. Int J Color Dis. 1994;9:77–81.
43. Beyer-Berjot L, Maggiori L, Birnbaum D, et al. A total laparoscopic approach reduces the infertility rate after ileal pouch-anal anastomosis: a 2-center study. Ann Surg. 2013;258:275–82.
44. Bartels SA, D'Hoore A, Cuesta MA, et al. Significantly increased pregnancy rates after laparoscopic restorative proctocolectomy: a cross-sectional study. Ann Surg. 2012;256:1045–8.
45. Hor T, Lefevre JH, Shields C, et al. Female sexual function and fertility after ileal pouch-anal anastomosis. Int J Color Dis. 2016;31:593–601.
46. Hjortswang H, Jarnerot G, Curman B, et al. The influence of demographic and disease-related factors on health-related quality of life in patients with ulcerative colitis. Eur J Gastroenterol Hepatol. 2003;15:1011–20.
47. Meijs S, Gardenbroek TJ, Sprangers MA, et al. Health-related quality of life and disability in patients with ulcerative colitis and proctocolectomy with ileoanal pouch versus treatment with anti-TNF agents. J Crohns Colitis. 2014;8:686–92.
48. Pinczowski D, Ekbom A, Baron J, et al. Risk factors for colorectal cancer in patients with ulcerative colitis: a case-control study. Gastroenterology. 1994;107:117–20.
49. Bernstein CN, Eaden J, Steinhart AH, et al. Cancer prevention in inflammatory bowel disease and the chemoprophylactic potential of 5-aminosalicylic acid. Inflamm Bowel Dis. 2002;8:356–61.
50. Sciaudone G, Pellino G, Riegler G, et al. Infliximab in drug-naive patients with failed ileorectal anastomosis for Crohn's disease: a new chance for sparing the rectum? Eur Surg Res. 2011;46:163–8.
51. Andersson P, Olaison G, Bodemar G, et al. Surgery for Crohn colitis over a twenty-eight-year period: fewer stomas and the replacement of total colectomy by segmental resection. Scand J Gastroenterol. 2002;37:68–73.
52. Andersson P, Olaison G, Hallböök O, et al. Segmental resection or subtotal colectomy in Crohn's colitis? Dis Colon Rectum. 2002;45:47–53.
53. Alessandroni L, Kohn A, Capaldi M, et al. Adenocarcinoma below stapled ileoanal anastomosis after restorative proctocolectomy for ulcerative colitis. Updat Surg. 2012;64:149–52.
54. Abdalla M, Landerholm K, Andersson P, et al. Risk of rectal cancer after colectomy for patients with ulcerative colitis-a national cohort study. Clin Gastroenterol Hepatol. 2017;15:1055–60. https://doi.org/10.1016/j.cgh.2016.11.036.

55. Uzzan M, Kirchgesner J, Oubaya N, et al. Risk of rectal neoplasia after colectomy and ileorectal anastomosis for ulcerative colitis. J Crohns Colitis. 2017;11(8):930–5.
56. Löffler T, Rossion I, Goossen K, et al. Hand suture versus stapler for closure of loop ileostomy-a systematic review and meta-analysis of randomized controlled trials. Langenbecks Arch Surg. 2015;400(2):193–205. https://doi.org/10.1007/s00423-014-1265-8.
57. Lepistö A, Järvinen HJ. Fate of the rectum after colectomy with ileorectal anastomosis in ulcerative colitis. Scand J Surg. 2005;94:40–2.
58. Tekkis PP, Heriot AG, Smith JJ, et al. Long-term results of abdominal salvage surgery following restorative proctocolectomy. Br J Surg. 2006;93:231–7.
59. Uzzan M, Cosnes J, Amiot A, et al. Long-term follow-up after Ileorectal anastomosis for ulcerative colitis: a GETAID/GETAID Chirurgie multicenter retrospective cohort of 343 patients. Ann Surg. 2017;266(6):1029–34. https://doi.org/10.1097/SLA.0000000000002022.
60. Landerholm K, Abdalla M, Myrelid P, et al. Survival of ileal pouch anal anastomosis constructed after colectomy or secondary to a previous ileorectal anastomosis in ulcerative colitis patients: a population-based cohort study. Scand J Gastroenterol. 2017;52:1–5.
61. Bulow S, Hojen H, Buntzen S, et al. Primary and secondary restorative proctocolectomy for familial adenomatous polyposis: complications and long-term bowel function. Color Dis. 2013;15:436–41.
62. Tulchinsky H, Cohen CR, Nicholls RJ. Salvage surgery after restorative proctocolectomy. Br J Surg. 2003;90:909–21.
63. Lovegrove RE, Tilney HS, Heriot AG, et al. A comparison of adverse events and functional outcomes after restorative proctocolectomy for familial adenomatous polyposis and ulcerative colitis. Dis Colon Rectum. 2006;49:1293–306.
64. Nordenvall C, Myrelid P, Ekbom A, et al. Probability, rate and timing of reconstructive surgery following colectomy for inflammatory bowel disease in Sweden: a population-based cohort study. Color Dis. 2015;17:882–90.
65. Block M, Jörgensen KK, Öresland T, et al. Colectomy for patients with ulcerative colitis and primary sclerosing cholangitis - what next? J Crohns Colitis. 2014;8:421–30.

# Chapter 15
# The Lived Experience

**Scott Clifford, Julia Spanswick, Kenny Graham, and Zarah Perry-Woodford**

**Abstract** A good outcome for the patient is, of course, one of the most desired aims when choosing to undergo ileal pouch surgery. Whilst an ileal pouch does not offer a return to normal bowel function, and is not without risk, it does offer many people an opportunity to return to life and the things they enjoy - after a period of illness or perhaps to mitigate further health complications which were previously invisible. Where a person is suitable for an ileal pouch they may opt for this as their surgical preference because it offers them not only an alternative to living with a stoma but a continent solution giving greater control over their bowel function, when compared to a stoma.

**Keywords** Patient experience · Personal journey · Patient outcomes · Support networks · Quality of life · Emotional considerations · The ileostomy and internal pouch support group (IA)

## 15.1 Introduction

The quality of life following ileoanal pouch surgery will however differ from person to person. Whilst success may be gauged by pouch function it is also important to remember that bowel surgery such as this can have an immeasurable effect on a person who may experience strong emotions before, during and after surgery. Emotions such as anger, frustration, embarrassment, fear or even relief, at the thought of 'being different' or the journey they have been through and the uncertainty of the one ahead. Dealing with these emotions can be difficult for some and whilst a patient will rely on their healthcare team for support, some feel as though you can only truly understand through personal experience.

S. Clifford · J. Spanswick · K. Graham
The Ileostomy and Internal Pouch Support Group (IA), National Office, Peverill House, Ballyclare, UK

Z. Perry-Woodford (✉)
St. Mark's Hospital, Harrow, UK
e-mail: zarah.perry-woodford@nhs.net

 
J. Warusavitarne, Z. Perry-Woodford (eds.), *The Ileoanal Pouch*,
https://doi.org/10.1007/978-3-319-94385-5_15

Of course not all outcomes are desirable and it is to be recognised that a percentage of pouches fail or do not function as intended, leaving a person with a poor experience which can impact their quality of life. Research continues to record patient experiences both in the short and long term following ileal pouch surgery and patient outcomes remain an important and decisive factor when a person is considering which route to take.

## 15.2 IA (The Ileostomy and Internal Pouch Support Group)

In 1956, IA (Ileostomy Association) was established and began supporting people living with an ileostomy. Through collaboration between patient and professional IA developed a network of support groups throughout the UK and Ireland. Using the experiences of others already living with an ileostomy, IA's visiting service quickly grew. Matching visitor to patient in terms of gender, age and lifestyle, IA found through experience that an IA visitor could help a person to move forward after surgery, either by offering practical day-to-day tips, or just talking as someone who had been through a similar experience.

In 1993, IA (The ileostomy and internal pouch Support Group) extended support to people living with an ileal pouch and now has a team of people solely representing the interests of those living with an ileal pouch.

With the important role that patient experience plays in determining outcome and the benefits that talking to someone who has been through a similar experience can offer, Julia and Kenny share their experience of living with debilitating illness leading to life with a stoma before surgery for an ileal pouch. Offering a view from both a male and female perspective, their journeys leading to pouch surgery are very different but address some of the important considerations that many are faced with when having bowel surgery; relationships, marriage, having a family and moving forward with pouch surgery knowing that uncertainty lies ahead.

## 15.3 Julia's Story

At 25, Julia started having problems with diarrhoea and blood in her stools; she was diagnosed with ulcerative colitis.

For 4 years she struggled with the disease - on and off steroid and other medication, spending periods of time in hospital to rest the bowel. As the number of stays increased so did the discussion around removal of her bowel. As time progressed she grew weaker and so did the number of visits to the toilet; Julia was now averaging 30 trips a day each time losing blood with each motion.

At 29 her health had deteriorated. She was put onto intravenous nutrition but was told that her colon had to be removed to save her life.

Devastated at the news that her colon was to be removed and that she would need an ileostomy, Julia told her fiancé how she would understand if he didn't want to stay with her. Julia felt she would be left looking like a freak. Looking back afterwards it seemed a crazy way to feel, but on the face of it, faced with the reality of surgery, it was how she felt. In the cold light of day, Julia knew she was losing her battle; attached to machines in hospital with her hair was falling out she knew one thing for certain. She didn't want to die.

Julia's fiancé was totally supportive and didn't care about the stoma. He just wanted her alive and in the best possible health so that she could walk down the aisle 9 months later – the wedding was already booked and he was determined it was going ahead!

Surgery quickly followed. Julia was given blood transfusions and vitamin injections in the meantime to try and build her up for surgery. On the day of surgery the stoma position was marked and down she went.

During her recovery after coming out of surgery it was her fiancé who saw my stoma first. Julia wasn't interested in looking at it, and recalls her words, "I don't want it, so I don't want to look at!"

It was suggested that Julia name her stoma, which some do after surgery as a way of helping with acceptance. She did think of one name for her stoma but it wasn't something welcoming or polite!

As time progressed in hospital she began to look at her stoma and was amazed at how it moved on its own! Eventually, with her thoughts together, she realised that surgery had saved her life, and that without 'Ruby', as she had now named her stoma, she wouldn't have made it.

Fast forward 9 months, Julia's hair had started to grow back, the big day had arrived and her outlook had changed dramatically. She was full of life and loving it. On her honeymoon, she was parascending off the back of a speed boat in Mauritius in a bikini (with a swim skirt) living life to the full and loved having control, which she hadn't had for a very long time when living with ulcerative colitis.

She ate everything and made sure she chewed her food well. On one occasion her stoma was blocked, caused by apple peel, but she carefully extracted the offending peel from her stoma.

With her rectum still in place, she continued to experience symptoms of colitis, and used suppositories to keep it calm. Julia's surgeon was keen for her to consider ileal pouch surgery but even in the short time with a stoma she was uncertain. Julia's family thought she was mad not to even consider getting rid of the bag, but ultimately it was her decision. Following discussions with her husband, they came to the conclusion that she had nothing to lose. Had pouch surgery been unsuccessful, at least she would know what life was like living with a stoma. Julia was now in a much stronger position compared to her previous surgery and felt her recovery would be much quicker.

Ileal pouch surgery was performed 1 year after losing her colon and she was given a loop stoma so the newly formed pouch could rest before being connected. Julia's experience with a loop stoma was, in her words, a nightmare and she suffered terrible burns to the skin around the stoma site, as it was a lot closer to her skin. On one occasion she recalls standing in the shower without a bag on letting warm water fall onto her stoma for relief, as she'd struggled to get a bag on. Thankfully her specialist nurse sorted out a bag for her to wear which helped tremendously, but after 3 months with the loop stoma she'd had enough and was pleased to welcome further surgery to close the loop stoma.

Early days with an ileal pouch were difficult for Julia. The frequency of trips to the toilet increased and were reminiscent of her days with colitis. Her bottom was sore from the frequency as it wasn't used to being wiped. Julia found comfort in Sudocrem which soothed the soreness and quickly became her friend! To increase her level of control in the pouch each time Julia had the urge to empty her pouch, she continued to hold her sphincter muscles in an attempt to train her pouch - and it worked. Julia is now emptying her pouch around 2–3 times a day, she rarely gets up during the night to empty and doesn't experience any leaks from the pouch. After taking advice from her surgical team, she started to regain her fitness gradually and undertook Pilates and other forms of exercise.

Throughout all this, Julia had one ambition. She wanted to become a mother and was unsure how her body would manage. After discussion with her surgeon, Julia started trying for a baby, and 8 months after surgery, she was pregnant. She felt so healthy. She had a great pregnancy although towards the end emptying the pouch became more difficult but her obstetrician kept a very close eye on progress, given the risk of complications.

It was decided that Julia would give birth by Caesarean section at 38 weeks to avoid any problems with the pouch and avoid damage to her sphincter muscles, leading to leakage or incontinence. During the birth, Julia's surgeon was on hand to check the pouch and ensure no damage had been sustained. Baby Isabella was born in the November and two and a half years later, Harry was born, again at 38 weeks by Caesarean section. Julia's second pregnancy was problem free.

In her own words, Julia describers her pouch as 'terrific' and she has great control. Although she has experienced narrowing in the end of her pouch and has had it stretched twice she now uses a Hegar dilator, under guidance from her medical team, twice a week to stop any future narrowing.

Julia is also no stranger to obstructions, caused by adhesions. After one surgery she was warned that she might have to return to living with a stoma and recalls what a welcome relief it was to wake up from surgery and find her pouch still intact.

Now following a low fibre and low residue diet after guidance from her medical team, she is grateful to have been 'obstruction-free' for a number of years now. It might not be for everyone but the measure of success living with an ileal pouch is a very individual thing and Julia feels a small price to pay to keep everything working fine.

Julia undertakes an exercise regime which includes bouncing up and down on a mini trampoline, but doesn't suffer any leaks. With regular Pilate's classes, Julia is also able to keep her core and mind strong.

Understandably nobody wants to have bowel surgery but Julia feels it has made her a stronger person. In the early days IA supported Julia through its visiting service and now, using her own experiences, Julia is now a visitor for IA herself.

## 15.4 Kenny's Story

In comparison to Julia, Kenny's experience is very different. His first experience of illness was back in 1991, just a few months after getting married. After falling unwell one evening and suffering violent sickness every hour or so, Kenny presented himself to the accident and emergency department. Following what was diagnosed as gastroenteritis, Kenny was sent home to drink plenty of fluids to recover.

This proved to be a turning point for his health and he started to notice an increase in trips to the toilet. His initial diagnosis was IBS and so on and off for the next 11 or 12 years, Kenny enjoyed periods of good health intertwined with what he describes as 'bowel problems.'

One particularly bad episode led to him being hospitalised in 2003 and a diagnosis of ulcerative colitis. Nine years followed, most it being good and only an occasional flare up where intravenous steroids quickly brought the inflammation under control. One particularly bad episode however, in 2012, was not so easy to manage and so surgery was recommended to avoid the bowel rupturing. Kenny recalls being left with very mixed emotions when being told this news. On one hand he was fearful of having surgery yet on the other he wondered if this was a path which would lead him to a life free from bowel problems.

Surgery was a success and despite having an ileostomy, Kenny's attitude was one of positivity at his newly found freedom to do what he wanted and when he wanted to do it. He'd already decided that further surgery to have an ileal pouch formed was what he wanted but for the time being he was in charge and was going to make the most of it! Kenny described it as long journey with a few low points but a journey that he was determined to win.

Away from his health issues Kenny has a great love of the countryside and living in Scotland has afforded him access to some of the most amazing scenery to be found in the world. He walked The West Highland Way (a 96 mile walk through the Highlands) with friends in 2002, just a year or so prior to being diagnosed with ulcerative colitis. It opened his eyes to some amazing scenery, particularly so when walking through Glencoe.

Following surgery in 2012, Kenny started climbing mountains again and completed several Munros (a Scottish mountain in excess of 3000 ft) as well as walking numerous other smaller hills and level walks.

His other main passion has always been music and has always enjoyed listening to artists such as Queen, Marillion and Pink Floyd to name a few of his favourites. With a new lease of life he felt more confident to travel both throughout the UK and Europe to enjoy some of his favourite artists.

Kenny has always known that further surgery was planned although as time passed his enthusiasm for having pouch surgery dwindled slightly since being free of colitis. In February 2016 however his ileal pouch was formed and he remained with a covering stoma. Surgery had taken over 6 h due to adhesions and his ensuing recovery was longer than anticipated. Two unfortunate bouts of paralytic ileus on two separate occasions only days apart during his recovery was difficult to cope with and he describes as 'one of his worst moments'. Following his recovery from ileus, 4 weeks after being discharged, Kenny suffered high output leading to dehydration. He was re-admitted to hospital and put onto a drip until he was well enough to return home.

Despite his setbacks and wanting to continue his enjoyment of the Scottish countryside, Kenny continued walking and going to concerts although on a reduced scale compared to before and at a much more leisurely rate.

His final procedure to close the stoma and put the pouch into function took place in September 2016 September and was by far the easiest of the three procedures. His recovery was much quicker and he was discharged after 7 days returning to work 5 days later. Thankfully his employer was understanding and so he was able to negotiate a working pattern that suited everyone whilst his recovery continued.

After four and a half years of living with a stoma Kenny had fully working bowel function again and although initially this was very frequent, things settled down relatively quickly to an emptying frequency of around about 5–6 times daily - a frequency that he had been informed was good so soon after surgery. As he became use to emptying the pouch he soon learned what foods led to soreness around the anal area, often referred to by patients as 'butt burn'; a condition typically due to undigested enzymes in the faecal waste coming through the pouch. Kenny also experienced another common issue for pouch patients knowing when there is wind to pass in the pouch and when there is not. Uncertainty can lead to leakage away from the toilet which can knock a person's confidence.

Like Julia, Kenny found benefit in talking to someone who had been through a similar experience before going through surgery himself. Kenny now uses his own experiences as an IA visitor to help others on their journey.

# Index


**A**
Abdominal pouch salvage, 82
Adenomatous polyposis coli (*APC*)
    tumour suppressor gene, 116
Afferent loop syndrome, 61, 62
Alicaforsen, 109, 110
Amitriptyline, 142
Anastomotic vaginal fistula, 66–67
Appendicostomy, 2

**B**
Biofeedback therapy
  in bowel dysfunction, 154
  evacuation techniques
    balloon expulsion, 156
    brace exercise, 156
    containment, 158
    neuromuscular stimulation, 157
    pelvic floor muscle exercises, 157
    pouch compliance training, 157
    psychological support, 158
    Qufora mini irrigation
      system, 157
    urge resistance training, 157
  and pouch function, 154
  at St Marks Hospital
    dietary modification, 156
    education, 155
    machine biofeedback therapy, 155
    pharmacotherapy, 155–156
    practical recommendations,
      154, 155
  therapeutic relationship, 154
B-pouch, 55
Brooke, B.N., 4

**C**
Cattell, R., 3
Close rectal dissection, 18, 50–51, 69, 85
Codeine phosphate, 142, 143
Cohen, Z., 9
Colectomy with ileorectal anastomosis, 5
Continent ileostomy, *see* Kock pouch
    procedure
Crohn's disease (CD), 68, 78, 85
  aetiology, 93
  complication rates, 92
  complications, 93
  diagnosis, 92
  differential diagnosis
    fistulating disease, 95
    pouch/ pre-pouch ileum, 94
    pouch-vaginal fistulae, 95
    small bowel obstruction, 95
    stricturing disease, 94
  histological findings, 92
  incidence of, 91
  management of
    fistulae, 97
    inflammation, 96
    pouch failure, 98
    pouch vaginal fistulae, 98, 99
    small bowel obstruction, 97
    strictures, 96, 97
  prognosis of, 99, 100
  symptoms, 92
Cuffitis, 67, 143

**D**
Defunctioning ileostomy, 11, 41, 52, 57, 65
Dioralyte®, 144




J. Warusavitarne, Z. Perry-Woodford (eds.), *The Ileoanal Pouch*,
https://doi.org/10.1007/978-3-319-94385-5

**E**
Efferent loop syndrome, 61, 63
Elective colectomies, 173
Emergency colectomies, 173
Endoanal flap advancements, 81
Enhanced recovery after surgery (ERAS) protocol, 53

**F**
*Faecalibacterium* spp., 108
  *F. prausnitzii*, 107
Familial adenomatous polyposis (FAP)
  *APC* tumour suppressor gene, 116
  clinical manifestations, 116–118
    benign extra-colonic manifestations, 117
    carcinomas, 117
    desmoids, 117
    gastrointestinal tract, 116, 117
    genotype-phenotype correlation, 118
  *de novo* germline mutation, 116
  desmoid disease, 123–125
  duodenal surveillance, 123
  flexible sigmoidoscopy, 123
  follow-up, 126–128
  laparoscopic/open surgery, 125–126
  *MutYH* gene, 116
  *POLE/POLD1 genes*, 116
  prevalence, 115
  RPC (*see* Restorative proctocolectomy (RPC))
  stapled IPAA, 126, 127
  surgical management
    completion proctectomy, 120
    pre-operative colonoscopy, 120
    rigid sigmoidoscopy, 120
    timing of surgery, 119
    total proctocolectomy, 120
  surveillance and diagnosis, 118, 119
Fazio, V.W., 8
Functional bowel disorders, 23–25

**G**
Gut microbiota, 106

**H**
Hegar dilators, 81, 147
H-pouch, 10
*Hyoscine butylbromide*, 143

**I**
Ileal pouch configurations, 9, 10
Ileal pouch-anal anastomosis (IPAA)
  disease factors
    Crohn's disease, 23
    indeterminate colitis, 22
    medical therapy, 22
    primary sclerosing colitis, 22
  for dysplasia/cancer, 18–20
  FAP, 126
  hand-sewn/stapled devices, 33, 34
  laparoscopic surgery, 23
  medical therapy, 22
  patient factors
    age, 20–21
    obesity, 21
  with proctocolectomy, 17
  reconstruction, 42 (*see also* Restorative proctocolectomy (RPC))
Ileoanal anastomosis, 2, 5–7, 10, 58, 68, 70
Ileorectal anastomosis
  anti-inflammatory medication, 178
  cancer risk, 178
  fecundability, 177
  functional outcome, 175–177
  high dose anti-inflammatory medication, 175
  maintenance therapy and surveillance algorithm, 178, 179
  quality of life, 178
  reconstructive algorithm, 180
  sexual function, 177
  surgical procedure, 175
  surgical risks and failure, 179, 181
The ileostomy and internal pouch Support Group, 188
IPAA, *see* Ileal pouch-anal anastomosis
Isotonic drinks, 144
Ispaghula Husk, 142

**J**
J-pouch, 9, 10, 56
  advantages, 55
  double stapled IPAA, 34
  evacuation issues, 32
  protective pads, 32
  short-term and long-term outcomes, 32
  two-limb J pouch, 32

**K**
Kock pouch procedure, 1, 6, 174, 175
  complications
    acute complications, 168
    fistula, 169
    Medena catheter draining, 168
    pouch leakage, 168
    stricturing, 169
    technical complications, 168
    valve problems and dislocation, 168–169
  contraindications, 163
  diagram of, 161, 162
  indications, 162–163
  long-term durability, 170
  nipple valve construction and fixation, 164–166
  post-operative care, 167
  pouch construction, 165, 166
  pouch posterior wall, measurement and construction, 164, 165
  quality of life, 170
  stoma formation and fixation, 166, 167

**L**
Lockhart Mummery, J.P., 2
Lomatil, 141
Loperamide, 141, 142

**M**
Machine biofeedback therapy, 155
Medena catheters, 37, 146, 147, 157
Miller, C.G., 3
Minimally invasive pouch surgery
  advantages, 45
  circular stapled anastomosis, 52
  closure of ileostomy, 53
  definition, 46
  ERAS protocol, 53
  evidence for, 47–48
  ileostomy formation, 52
  operating room set up, 47, 48
  patient positioning, 46
  patient selection, 46
  port placement, 46, 49
  port positioning, 46
  port set up, 46, 49
  pouch formation, 51
  single stapled anastomosis, 51
  specimen extraction, 51
  subtotal colectomy, 49
  trans-anal proctectomy, 51
Mucosectomy, 55

**N**
Nicholls, R.J., 7
Nissen, R., 5

**O**
Oresland, T., 8

**P**
Panproctocolectomy, 17, 19
Parc, R., 8
Parks, A.G., 6
Pelvic floor muscle exercises, 157
PNP, *see* Pouch nurse practitioner
Polyposis syndromes, 7, 116
Pouch configurations
  evacuation issues, 32
  four-limb W pouch, 32
  hand-sewn/stapled devices, 33, 34
  protective pads, 32
  quality of life, 33
  three-limb S pouch, 32
  two-limb J pouch, 32
Pouch dislocation, 37
Pouch failure
  causes of, 76
  Crohn's disease, 98
  diagnosis, 76
  pelvic abscess, 86
  postoperative complication, 84
  pouch salvage surgery, 76, 78
    chronic presacral abscess cavity, 80
    clinical manifestations, 79
    clinicopathological conditions, 78
    Crohn's disease, 85
    indications, 76, 77
    local/perineal salvage, 79
    median bowel frequency, 86
    patient satisfaction rates, 86
    pouch stenosis, 84
    redo salvage, 79, 80
    revisional salvage, 79, 80
    success rates, 84
    treatment outcomes, 78, 82

Pouch failure (*cont.*)
with pouch-vaginal fistulas, 85
quality of life, 76
redo ileal pouch surgery, 77
risk of, 148
treatment, 148
Pouch lengthening techniques
anterior and posterior mesenteric incisions, 39
apex variation, 42
bowstring excision, 41, 42
hand sewn anastomosis, 43
key steps, 38
pouch folding, 43
small bowel mesentery mobilisation, 39
S-shaped pouch, 43
vascular division, 39–41
vascular supply, 38
Pouch microbiota, 106, 107
Pouch nurse practitioner (PNP)
complications
abdominal and anal pain, 143
bowel obstructions, 144
cuffitis, 143
dehydration, 144
anal fissure, 148
incomplete evacuation, 145, 146
increased frequency and urgency, 141, 142
leakage and seepage, 142
pouch anal anastomotic stricture misdiagnosis, 146, 148
pouchitis, 142
contraception, 135
dietary advice, 137, 138
fertility and fecundity, 134
follow up, 139, 140
medication advice, 140, 141
nurse-led pouch clinic, 139
perianal skin care, 137, 138
post-operative care, 136
pregnancy and delivery, 135
pre-operative counselling, 131, 132
pre-operative factors, 133
rehydration fluids, 144
sexual function, 133, 134
sexuality, 133, 134
stoma care, 136
stoma closure, 137
Pouch prolapse, 64, 65, 81
Pouch salvage surgery, 76
chronic presacral abscess cavity, 80
clinical manifestations, 79
clinicopathological conditions, 78
Crohn's disease, 85
indications, 76, 77
local/perineal salvage, 79
median bowel frequency, 86
patient satisfaction rates, 86
pouch stenosis, 84
redo salvage, 79, 80
revisional salvage, 79, 80
success rates, 84
treatment outcomes, 78, 82
Pouchitis, 32
antibiotic induced remission, 106
antibiotic treatment, 109
bacterial analysis, 107
bacterial diversity, 107, 108
biologic drugs, 109
complications, 143
diagnosis, 106
flexible pouchoscopy, 108
immunosuppressants, 109
incidence of, 106
maintenance therapy, 110, 111
microbiota, 107
and non-pouchitis groups, 107
NSAIDS, 143
oral budesonide, 109
pathogenesis of, 106
suphasalzine treatment, 109
treatment, 106
TRFLP technique, 107
video capsule endoscopy, 109
Pre-pouch ileitis (PPI), 92, 108–110
Primary sclerosing colitis (PSC), 22
Proctocolectomy, 15
without ileostomy, 6
with permanent ileostomy, 4
*See also* Restorative proctocolectomy (RPC)
Proteobacteria, 106–108

**Q**

Qufora mini irrigation system, 157

**R**

Redo pouch surgery, 76
complications, 83
integral components, 80
operative indications, 77
permanent end-ileostomy, 80
for pouch-vaginal fistulas, 81
quality of life, 86
short-term complications, 83
success rates, 84

Restorative proctocolectomy (RPC), 131
- clinical results, 7, 9
- Crohn's disease (*see* Crohn's disease (CD))
- dysfunction, septic causes of
  - anastomotic vaginal fistula, 66, 67
  - Crohn's disease, 68
  - cuffitis, 67
  - presacral sinus, 64–67
  - retained rectum, 68
- early complications, 58–60
- familial adenomatous polyposis, 6
- FAP
  - prophylactic surgery, 121, 122
  - sphincter-sparing surgery, 120
- for functional bowel disorders, 24
- late pouch dysfunction, 60
- mechanical causes of dysfunction
  - afferent loop, 63
  - afferent loop syndrome, 61, 62
  - anastomotic stricture, 61
  - efferent loop syndrome, 61
  - pouch prolapse, 64, 65
  - redundant blind loop, 64
  - torsion of pouch, 63
- modified two stage, 57
- one stage, 56
- pouch nurse practitioner (*see* Pouch nurse practitioner (PNP))
- rectal cancer, 120
- surgical approaches
  - cuff/efferent loop excision, 68, 69
  - redo operations, 71
  - retained rectum, 69, 70
- three stage, 57
- two stage, 57
- for ulcerative colitis, 6

**S**

S pouch, 9, 43, 56
- short-term and long-term outcomes, 32
- three-limb S pouch, 32

Single-incision laparoscopic surgery (SILS), 11
St. Mark's Hospital Electrolyte Mix, 144, 145
Stapled ileoanal J-pouch reservoir, 56
Surgical Committee of the European Crohn's and Colitis Organisation (S-ECCO) guidelines, 57

**T**

Tension-free pouch-anal anastomosis, 38
Terminal restriction fragment length polymorphism (T-RFLP), 106, 107
Transanal minimally invasive surgery (TAMIS), 11, 57, 67
Transanal proctectomy pouch, 35

**U**

Ulcerative colitis (UC), 17
- acute, 16, 17
- appendicostomy, 2
- case study, 188–192
- definition, 15
- elective setting, 17
- intractability, 17
- IPAA (*see* Ileal pouch anal anastomosis (IPAA))
- mortality rate, 2
- natural history of, 15
- proctocolectomy, 15
  - without ileostomy, 6
  - with permanent ileostomy, 4

Utsunomiya, J., 10

**W**

W pouch, 10, 56
- four-limb W pouch, 32
- short-term and long-term outcomes, 32

MIX
Papier aus verantwortungsvollen Quellen
Paper from responsible sources
FSC® C105338

If you have any concerns about our products,
you can contact us on
**ProductSafety@springernature.com**

In case Publisher is established outside the EU,
the EU authorized representative is:
**Springer Nature Customer Service Center GmbH**
**Europaplatz 3, 69115 Heidelberg, Germany**

Printed by Libri Plureos GmbH
in Hamburg, Germany